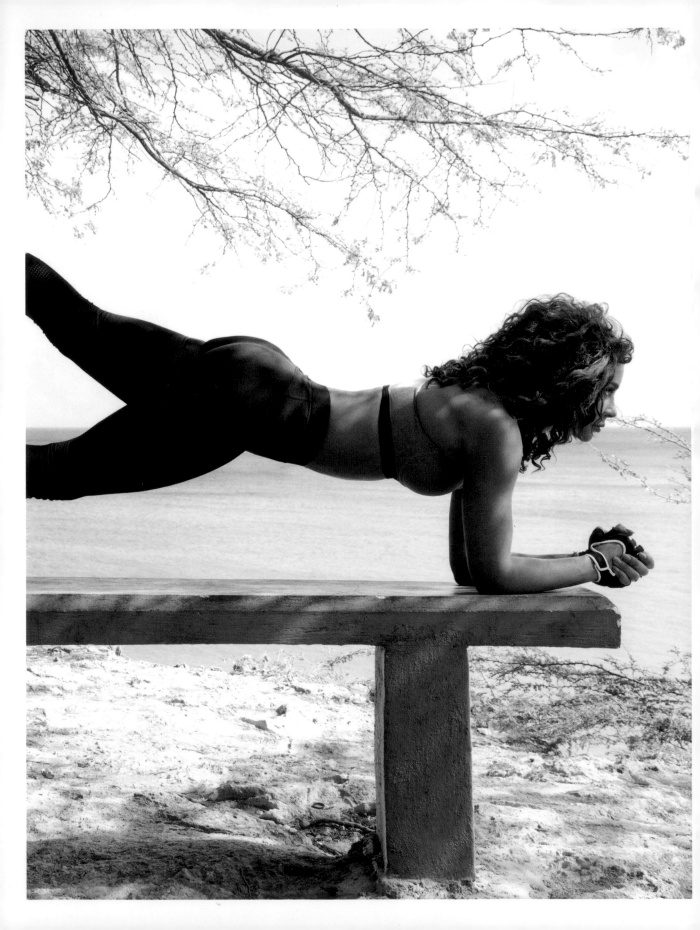

Fajah Lourens

THE KILLERBODY PLAN

Recipes and workouts to get lean in 12 weeks

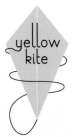

yellow
kite

#mkbm #killerbodydiet
#killerbodychallenge

 /mykillerbodymotivation

 @mykillerbodymotivation

First published in the Netherlands in 2016
by Kosmos Uitgevers

First published in Great Britain in 2016 by Yellow Kite

An imprint of Hodder & Stoughton

An Hachette UK company

1

Copyright © Fajah Lourens 2016

Cover and interior design: Autobahn

Photographs on pages 2, 31, 71, 76, 165 and front cover: Martika de Sanders

Food photography on pages 38, 166–193: Frans Schreurs

Photography on pages 39, 44, 68, 194–203 and back cover (left): Sven ter Heide

Photography on page 7: Alexander Popelier

Photography on pages 112–146 and back cover (right): Rob Woo

Illustrations on pages 22–23: Sam Looman

Text in cooperation with: Anke Langelaan, Nanneke Schreurs, Daphne Groothuyse

Advanced schedules for diet and training: Wesley van Staveren

A CIP catalogue record for this title is available from the British Library

Trade paperback ISBN 978 1 473 65347 4

Ebook ISBN 978 1 473 65348 1

The advice herein is not intended to replace the services of trained health and fitness professionals, or be a substitute for medical advice. You are advised to consult with your health care professional with regards to matters relating to your health, and in particular regarding matters that may require diagnosis or medical attention.

Printed and bound in Germany by Firmengruppe Appl

Hodder & Stoughton policy is to use papers that are natural, renewable and recyclable products and made from wood grown in sustainable forests. The logging and manufacturing processes are expected to conform to the environmental regulations of the country of origin.

Yellow Kite, an imprint of Hodder & Stoughton Ltd
Carmelite House
50 Victoria Embankment
London EC4Y 0DZ

www.yellowkitebooks.co.uk
www.hodder.co.uk

Contents

6
Motivation

Welcome to The Killerbody Plan. The photos in this book and on all of my #MKBM social media tell a story of **success**, and it's a story that makes me really happy and proud! I've worked very hard to get to where I am today though, and it has taken a lot of **self-discipline**. My journey hasn't exactly been glamorous, quite the opposite in fact! But I hope it shows you how you can turn those negatives into **positives**. THE KILLER BODY PLAN will **motivate** and **help** you, especially when you're not in a good place to start with – always remember, I wasn't either. But **if I can do it, so can you!**

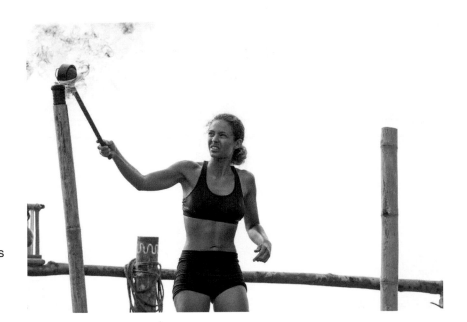

Four years ago, the Dutch children's charity the CliniClowns Foundation invited me to take part in the New York marathon. I was doing hardly any exercise or sport at the time and it seemed like a great opportunity to get back into it. My previous enthusiastic endeavours had all failed within the first three months and been followed by equally enthusiastic binge-eating, so to me the marathon seemed the perfect way to show myself I did have perseverance. *If it takes me a whole year to prepare for this, I will surely keep it up afterwards* – or so I thought.

Having zero running experience, I had to start completely from scratch. Fortunately, after sticking at it for a few weeks, I realised I was in fact doing much better than I'd thought. But then, just when I had managed to run 11 miles, I got a surprise invitation to take part in the Dutch version of the *Survivor* game show, *Expedition Robinson*. It turned out another contestant had pulled out at the last minute and I was asked to take their place. I accepted, with only two weeks to prepare!

The idea of the TV show is that you're essentially stranded on a desert island so I thought all the swimming would keep up my fitness levels . . . but I clearly had no idea what

was in store. I actually made it to the final (still so proud!), but it had taken five weeks of extreme physical exertion on very little food. Once I got home it was back to square one; all my fitness was gone, my body was in a state of shock. I had lost 11 kilos (24 lbs) in just over a month but now I was gaining 1 kilo back every day. My body started to hold on to everything I ate, and my eating habits were out of control. I had been dreaming of food all the way through the programme and now that it was possible to eat again there was no holding me back! I was indiscriminate in what I fancied, and what I fancied I ate.

To make things worse, I now only had 3 months to go before the New York marathon and an extremely heavy training schedule ahead of me.

If there was one thing I didn't fancy doing, it was running. Having just returned from a 33-day stint on an island, I was, in fact, in need of a break. Unfortunately, there was no time for that so I spent the next few months trying to build up my energy levels to run 34 miles a week. That made me very hungry indeed but no problem, I thought, with all that training I was doing I should eat well, and so I did. The result: a lot of cellulite and fat. I think I must have been the first person ever to become fat and flabby by training for a marathon.

In hindsight, knowing what I know now through #MKBM, it is hardly surprising that things got so bad. Running such long distances stimulates production of the stress hormone cortisol, which makes your body store fat. I was also eating a lot of soya products; soya stimulates production of oestrogen, which causes extra fat to be stored in the legs and this is what causes cellulite. Moreover, I was eating far more than I was burning off and, thanks to the *Expedition Robinson* experience, my body held on to everything I put into it. Conclusion: I looked a mess. And just when I thought things couldn't get any worse, I injured my knee just before I was supposed to leave for New York and was prescribed painkillers. Then, to top it all, the marathon was cancelled. Well, what can I say . . . I've certainly learned from that experience!

It was at that point, in 2012, that I realised it was time to turn my life around. First, I decided to post a photo of myself – a 'before' – on Instagram, because I knew that it would force me to post an 'after' photo as well –

exactly the push I needed. And I can tell you now, it worked! I am fit, I am happy and those rare occasions when I feel the urge to binge on food last no longer than a few hours. Better still, my healthy lifestyle is inspiring other people. It's amazing!

Introduction

Fantastic, well done for getting this book! It's the first step to a killer body!

The great thing about THE KILLER BODY PLAN is that you can use it in so many different ways. Perhaps you want to lose weight, or build muscle, or maybe you just want to start eating more healthily. Regardless of your personal motivation and your ideas about a killer body, this book will give you all the information to achieve your goal – at long last! This introduction gives the overview and key points, and I will go into these in more detail in the following chapters. I hope it will help you achieve that killer body. Let's go for it!

Goals

The first step in achieving your goals is defining exactly what they are. Do that right at the start. Jot down your current weight and measurements, take a picture of yourself, and do this every two weeks initially.

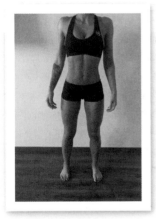

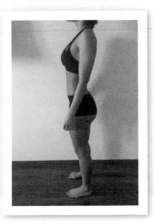

This is a really effective way of keeping track of your progress, which is such an important part of the process! A mirror won't show you the difference but the photos will, giving you a much-needed boost when you're finding it hard to keep motivated.

Dieting

You will find two types of diets in this book: the slimming diet, which consists of 3 phases, and the sports diet. We will stick to each phase for one month: so one month following the Phase 1 diet, then one month on Phase 2, and finally one month on Phase 3 – 12 weeks in total. Then, if you have achieved your goals in those three months, the next step will be making sure you maintain that weight (see page 46).

Here's a handy tip from the offset: sticking to the Phase 1 diet, a healthy balance of protein, fat, vegetables, fruit and moderate carbohydrates, will help you control your weight for the rest of your life. While you are following the diet, you will eat fewer calories than you really need each day, but once you have reached your target weight you can gradually increase the calories to the amount you require. I will explain how you can calculate your personal daily calorie needs later on in the book.

If by the end of the 12 weeks you haven't achieved your target weight and you have more than 24% body fat (a healthy average target), you should go back to Phase 1 or 2. If your body fat percentage is lower but you haven't quite achieved the goals you set, then continue with Phase 3.

The sports diet is only for people who have less than 24% body fat, and those who are very active; it does not follow on from the slimming diet.

To complement the diets, I have compiled a varied list of foods. If you are intolerant to or would rather not eat a certain kind of food, you can always swap it for a suitable alternative from that list. But remember, you should only swap fats for fats and protein for another protein: never substitute fat for protein.

EXAMPLE

Instead of white fish, you can eat chicken if you prefer. But you can't replace chicken with an avocado, for instance, because an avocado is mainly fat and chicken is mainly protein.

'ALL YOU NEED IS A SKIPPING ROPE, A CHAIR AND A PIECE OF ELASTIC'

The home exercises should be done at least three days a week, but you can do them as often as you like. So you could do an extra day of the same exercises, or carry on with your usual sports activities on the other days.

Training

The book also gives a choice of three different training phases, which you can just as easily do at home. All you need is a skipping rope, a chair and a piece of elastic. Like the diet phases, each phase lasts for four weeks. So after a month you will be ready for Phase 2. If you work out at the gym a lot, this book will give you various routines that you can do over two-, three-, four- or five-day sessions. It is up to you what schedule you follow, depending on how often you normally work out, and obviously you can decide for yourself what days to train. The possibilities are endless!

Setbacks

It's now been three years since I started my healthy-living regime, but you'd be wrong to assume I've never had a setback in all that time. There have been several occasions where, after allowing myself a 'just-this-once' treat, I actually carried on eating that way for two weeks, and one time when I really let myself go for a whole month. Obviously, I know now that when you're not working out you should eat less, but somehow, I seem to eat more when things get in the way of my training. Does that sound familiar to you too?

I have since learned to take control when I start to feel gluttonous, and fortunately those moods are now few and far between.

'THAT TINY BIT OF CHOCOLATE IS A HURDLE TO YOUR SUCCESS'

Whenever I need to get a grip, I ask myself: why do you let yourself go like this? Because if you know why you are doing something, you can prevent it more easily. For me, the reason is often that I am not happy in my own skin or I am upset about something that has happened.

Chocolate then seems like a godsend, but how long does the taste actually last? You can come up with all the silly excuses to justify eating that piece of chocolate: 'That tiny little piece won't make any difference, I am always at the gym, I have earned it. Tomorrow's another day, I'll just start afresh', and so on.

But that tiny little piece really does make a difference because it is a hurdle to achieving your goal.

What always helps me is that 'before' photo I have on my phone, of me when I started #MKBM; when I am about to give in, looking at that picture reminds me I do not want to look like that again, and that is all the motivation I need. And when I'm not feeling so happy? I find listening to good music helps!

Planning your treats

Although you should never indulge too much, you can have a sweet treat now and again – life would be very dull without them. But the key is to plan the treat moments because temptation is everywhere: a piece of birthday cake, a biscuit to go with your coffee, it all adds to your daily sugar intake. Sometimes you just pop that biscuit into your mouth

without a second thought and hey presto, another 80 calories that will take half an hour of power training at the gym to get rid of. So choose your treat moments wisely – you will actually enjoy them all the more for it.

Cheat meal

Once you get past the first 12 weeks, you can plan one cheat meal every week; write it down in your diary. Not a whole cheat day, mind, just one cheat meal. But do remember that if you are still trying to lose weight it is really important that you stay below your daily calorie needs at all times, and don't kid yourself: 'I've stuck to my diet for five days now, so I'll just ease up a bit over the weekend.' That is not how it works. While you are striving to achieve your killer body shape, stick to the diet seven days a week, and only allow yourself one cheat meal per week *after* those first 12 weeks.

If you can manage without a cheat meal altogether, I would advise you to do so until your body fat percentage has dropped significantly, in the last four weeks of dieting. But a lot of people find this very hard (so don't feel guilty) and need something to look forward to. If you happen to be one of those, you can choose to have a treat like a cake or some chocolate once a week. Trust me, it will not make you fat, but do be aware it will just take that little bit longer to reach your goal. So all the better if you can manage without!

'ONCE YOU GET PAST THE FIRST 12 WEEKS, PLAN ONE CHEAT MEAL EVERY WEEK'

Saboteurs

We all know them, those people who try to bring you down, saying things like, 'Oh, one biscuit won't hurt, will it?' or 'Are you not having a drink? That's so boring' or 'Wow, that's a lot of fuss, bringing your own food, I don't think I could be bothered' or 'But you're not fat' or 'You're taking this too far, why don't you try having some fun!' I call them saboteurs. Often lacking the willpower to lose weight or work out, they make themselves feel better by trying to persuade you to join them, to just have that little glass of wine, so that you will fail as well. If you have friends like that, be prepared. If you are going out, to a party or a work do perhaps, and you know you may be tempted, make sure you are not hungry and always take your own food wherever you go, ignoring those who criticise you for it. What matters is that you know why you are doing it. Never be persuaded to have just that one little drink or snack if it is not part of your plan. Be strong, you can do it! It will get easier once you have read this book!

I

SETTING GOALS

You are now
ready to start THE
KILLER BODY PLAN! We
will be setting some **tough** but
realistic targets, and I'll tell you
how to achieve them by adopting
a **healthy lifestyle** that combines
rigorous exercise with a **balanced
diet**. This is simply the safest and
most effective way to achieve
– and, moreover, keep –
your killer body.

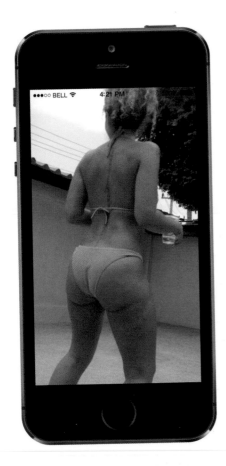

BEFORE

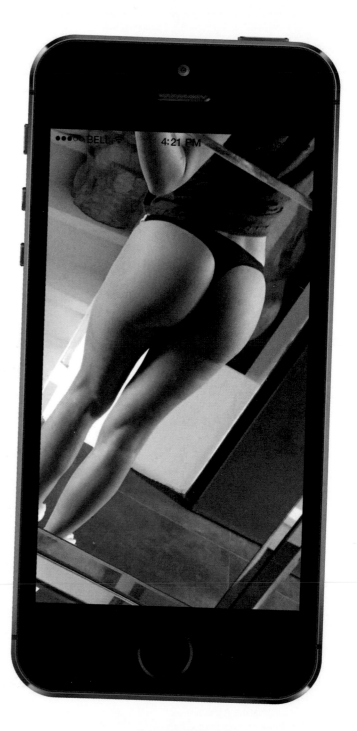

AFTER

I'm not going to lie: sticking to the strict exercise and diet regime will not always be easy. It can be extremely demanding both physically and mentally, and will take a lot of time and effort. As a working mother of two, I know only too well how disciplined you have to be to set the time aside. But don't give yourself any excuses: get your priorities straight. I get up at 6.30 a.m. to do my exercises, so that I am ready for my children when their day starts. There is no getting around it: you will have to make sacrifices to get a killer body. That last M in #MKBM really does stand for Motivation!

Obviously it is entirely up to you how rigidly you follow the 12-week diet and exercise regime. I have no control over whether you do or don't. But I promise that if you do, the results will start to show after only three weeks. You will feel inspired to carry on, and start to find it easier to meet the mental challenge of staying with it.

TIP

Take a picture of yourself every 2–4 weeks, just to chart your own progress, if anything. Posting them on social media using my #MKBM hashtag might give you the external pressure you need, knowing that people may comment if you haven't posted anything for a while (which could lead them to believe you have actually given up). You could even go as far as to ask your friends to keep track, if you think that might help. The many positive reactions I have received have certainly kept me going these last few years!

'DON'T GIVE YOURSELF ANY EXCUSES: GET YOUR PRIORITIES STRAIGHT'

At the very least, take your measurements every four weeks: hips, waist, belly and arms, just so you can monitor your own progress towards the ultimate goal, and assess whether you need to adjust your training or diet regime. The added benefit is that you will also be able to notice changes in your body shape straight away and I can't emphasise this enough: results = motivation. It will help you to stick with it when you are finding it all a bit of a struggle.

But let's get back to the start. We can't start working towards a goal if we haven't even defined it yet, so that is the first step in the process. Bear in mind that your goal must be realistic for you personally, which depends on your situation: what is your body type and your current regime? Are you active or have you done no exercise for a long time?

To get the full picture, which will serve as the basis for deciding on the right diet and exercise plan for you, you should answer the following questions.

My killer body chart

	AT THE START	AFTER 2 WEEKS
WEIGHT		
WAIST		
HIPS		
RIGHT THIGH		
LEFT THIGH		
RIGHT ARM		
LEFT ARM		

	AFTER **4** WEEKS	AFTER **6** WEEKS
WEIGHT		
WAIST		
HIPS		
RIGHT THIGH		
LEFT THIGH		
RIGHT ARM		
LEFT ARM		

AFTER **8** WEEKS   AFTER **10** WEEKS

WEIGHT

WAIST

HIPS

RIGHT THIGH

LEFT THIGH

RIGHT ARM

LEFT ARM

AFTER **12** WEEKS

WEIGHT

WAIST

HIPS

RIGHT THIGH

LEFT THIGH

RIGHT ARM

LEFT ARM

What is my body type?

A *Ectomorph*   **B** *Mesomorph*   **C** *Endomorph*

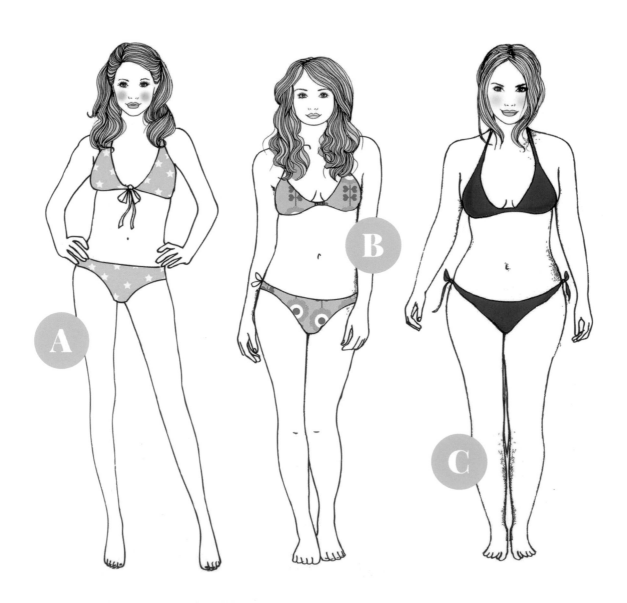

Before taking on the Killer Body challenge it is important that you know your body type, as this will determine the most effective exercise and diet regime for you. It would be a shame if you looked in the mirror only to conclude that all your efforts had gone to waste, wouldn't it? So take a closer look at your body, focusing on three aspects: your shape, size and frame.

Obviously no two bodies are the same, but the various combinations of these aspects are said to make three basic body types: ectomorph, mesomorph and endomorph.

Sounds a bit scientific (I didn't think of these, it's a theory devised by an American psychologist called Dr William H. Sheldon in the 1940s), but they are really quite easy to identify. Endomorph is basically the term for someone who is overweight, mesomorph describes someone who is muscular, while the ectomorph has neither a lot of fat nor muscle. Next, I will go into each of these three types in a little more detail.

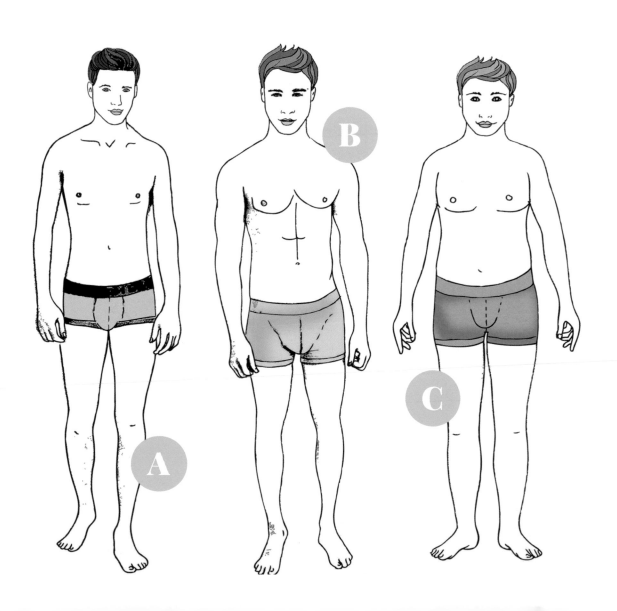

The ectomorph body type

The ectomorph tends to have a slim build and narrow frame, and struggles to gain weight and muscle. People who have this body type are often very suited to endurance sports such as running marathons.

KEY CHARACTERISTICS

- Narrow shoulders and hips
- Narrow face, high forehead
- Skinny legs, arms, small chest and flat stomach
- Smaller and weaker joints
- Dry muscle mass and very little body fat
- Difficulty gaining weight
- Very high metabolism

It is much more difficult for an ectomorph to gain and maintain muscle mass. Nevertheless, with the right training and diet plan you can still develop a killer body!

TRAINING FOR THE ECTOMORPH BODY TYPE

Frequency
Your training should focus on 1 or 2 muscle groups at a time, for example one big muscle group (your chest, legs or back) or two smaller muscle groups (biceps, triceps, hamstrings, calves, abs or shoulders). Each muscle group should be worked at least once a week, but make sure you get plenty of rest between training sessions, and never exercise muscles that are still sore from the last time you worked them. You should also change your training routine every 4 to 6 weeks, increasing or changing the weights you use each time. Remember to work hard, but only for short stints.

Sets/Repetitions
Raise the benchmark by doing compound exercises, otherwise known as multi-joint exercises, which work one or more muscle groups and multiple joints. This ensures that:

- The deeper muscle fibres are also exercised
- More calories are burned
- You train your whole body much faster
- Your coordination, reaction times and balance improve
- The stability and balance of opposing muscles surrounding your joints improve
- The risk of injury is reduced
- Your heart rate remains high
- Your muscles do not tire as quickly so you can train for longer
- You can lift heavier weights and so build more strength

Repeat 5–10 times, 6–8 sets per muscle group, but make sure you don't overdo it because that can actually impede muscle gain.

Intensity/Volume
Use heavier weights to increase intensity, but rest for at least 60 seconds between sets and for at least 5 minutes between exercising different parts of the body. You can use intensity techniques now and again if you like, but don't rely on them too much. Some examples:

- Forced repetitions: if you can no longer carry on, get someone else to help you do the last few repetitions, until you are able to carry on by yourself.
- Supersets: two exercises in quick succession with no break in between, i.e. one set of the first exercise, put the weights down and immediately start the second exercise set.
- Tri-sets: three different exercises carried out one after the other without a break in between.

Recuperation/Recovery
Longer recovery times mean more rest days need to be taken. Ectomorphs have a high metabolism and therefore need at least eight hours sleep, and if possible a nap during the day. Never train when you are tired or have not fully recuperated from your last session.

Aerobics/Cardio
Keep cardio activity to a minimum; certainly no more than 3 times a week. Too much aerobic exercise can actually decrease muscle gain, so make your training low-intensity and exercise no longer than 20 minutes per session.

DIET FOR THE ECTOMORPH BODY TYPE
A healthy, balanced diet and good supplements are essential. Eat 5 to 7 small meals per day (including drinks for weight gain), every 2.5 to 3 hours. Avoid sugars, especially the simple or fast sugars in liquorice, soft drinks, snack bars, biscuits, cake, sweets, fruit juices and ice cream. Do eat low-glycaemic index foods (a measure that indicates how quickly carbohydrates are broken down into glucose in the blood) such as beans, corn, sweet potatoes, oats, pasta, brown rice and wholemeal foods. Have 1 multivitamin and mineral drink and at least 2.5 litres of water a day, as well as a protein shake 90 minutes before bed.

The mesomorph body type

Mesomorphs tend to be athletic, muscular and lean, and have good posture. It is more or less the 'perfect' body type, making the rest of us quite envious. They have little trouble losing fat and gaining muscle, and are hardly ever under- or overweight. Life can be so unfair!

KEY CHARACTERISTICS

- Large head, broad shoulders and narrow waist (wedge shape)
- Muscular body, strong forearms and thighs
- Very low body fat
- Genetically blessed, highest bodybuilding potential
- Long torso, full chest, good shoulder-to-waist ratio

People with this body type can pretty much eat what they like and skip the gym now and again without it having any visible impact on their muscularity. It is Mother Nature's wonderful gift to them: being able to eat and train whichever way they please. Still, if they want to have a killer body, they too will have to be disciplined and work very hard!

TRAINING FOR THE MESOMORPH BODY TYPE

Frequency

The mesomorph body type responds well to intensive training, combining compound exercises (working multiple joints) with isolation exercises (working only one joint at a time). The more varied the training, the better the results will be in terms of muscle gain. Change the intensity of your workout every 3 to 4 weeks (high vs low), to promote growth and strength and avoid burnout.

Sets/Repetitions

Do explosive compound exercises using heavy weights (to improve your strength), before finishing off with isolation exercises. For most of the muscle groups you should repeat the exercises 8–12 times. But don't overdo it because, in spite of popular belief, more training does not build muscle any faster.

Intensity/Volume

Mesomorphs should keep their body alert by regularly changing training intensity, fitness exercises, sets, repetitions, weights and rests. It will also help to frequently interchange light, medium and heavy training days, and to combine slow and fast repetitions.

Recuperation/Recovery

The mesomorph may have a natural advantage, but it is still vitally important to rest so as not to actually impede muscle gain. Sleeping 7–9 hours a night is highly recommended, and obviously you should not train any parts of the body that have not yet fully recovered. An extra day of rest when you lack the energy, motivation or strength will certainly not do any harm.

Aerobics/Cardio

For the strongest muscle growth, 3 20–30-minute cardio training sessions per week are the maximum, i.e. a 5-minute warm-up, a 15–20 minute cardio exercise, followed by another 5-minute cooldown.

DIET FOR THE MESOMORPH BODY TYPE

Eat various low-fat, high-protein foods, such as chicken without the skin, turkey, eggs, lean beef and (white) fish. Drink at least 2.5 litres of water per day. Try not to do too much too soon, which could easily cause injuries or burnout. Listen to your body and be patient but persistent.

The endomorph body type

Endomorphs are often described as 'beefy' or heavy-set. They tend to have a soft, round body, a broad frame and find it hard to lose weight. Although dry training and losing fat are a struggle, they can gain muscle quite quickly.

KEY CHARACTERISTICS

- Wide hips and narrow shoulders (pear shape)
- A lot of fat across the whole body, including upper arms and thighs
- Small ankles and wrists, unfortunately accentuating the larger size of other parts of the body
- A broad frame
- Slow metabolism
- Gains weight easily, slow to lose fat
- Tendency to store fat

Endomorphs need a strict diet and a lot of exercise. Smaller meals, several times a day, are key.

TRAINING FOR THE ENDOMORPH BODY TYPE

Frequency
The endomorph needs to train often, especially aerobic exercises (long duration, so that it increases heart rate and breathing). Do 3 to 5 exercises for each muscle group, starting with the abs. Interchange full body routines (training your whole body) with a split-routine (only a few muscle groups). The purpose of the training is to increase metabolism and reduce body fat. Do not be afraid to experiment; variation is good for this body type and the only way to find out what suits you personally.

Sets/Repetitions
Do mainly high-intensity training, using moderate weights and taking minimal breaks in between the sets. Never do more than 8 sets per body part, though. Repeat exercises for the upper body 9–12 times, and exercises for the legs and calves 12–25 times.

Intensity/Volume
High-intensity training like iso-tension or continuous tension (tensing your muscles for shorter or longer), supersets, tri-sets and giant sets (2, 3 or a whole series of exercises in a row, no rests in between) will promote maximum muscle gain. During the last set of exercises focusing on a specific body part, use drop-sets (i.e. do it several

times, decreasing the weight as you go along).

Recuperation/Recovery
Train regularly but ensure that you leave at least 48 hours between training the same muscle group. As endomorphs have a slower metabolism, they do not need to sleep quite as much; in principle 7.5 hours should be sufficient.

Aerobics/Cardio
Cardio exercises are a very important part of training for an endomorph. You will burn relatively more fat doing low- to medium-intensity training, and by avoiding high-impact exercises that put a lot of stress on the joints. Cardio training should be done 3 times a week for at least 30 minutes, of which 20 minutes should be in your 'heart rate zone' (this is always under the maximum heart rate, but you can ask a personal trainer how to work this out for you personally), a 5-minute warm-up and 5-minute cool-down.

DIET FOR THE ENDOMORPH BODY TYPE

Endomorphs should follow a low-fat diet, containing only low-fat dairy products and various low-fat proteins. Avoid evening snacks or if you can't, eat something healthy at least. It is vital that you count your daily calorie intake. Do not drink anything containing sugar and/or alcohol, but do drink a lot of water (at least 2.5 litres a day).

II
NUTRITION

People often think that
losing weight is just a matter
of exercising more and eating less.
If only it was that simple. Losing
weight sensibly and effectively and
maintaining a killer body to boot is
a bit more demanding. What will make
the difference is a healthy, balanced
diet: you can train till you drop,
but without the right nutrition
your personal goals will always
be out of reach.

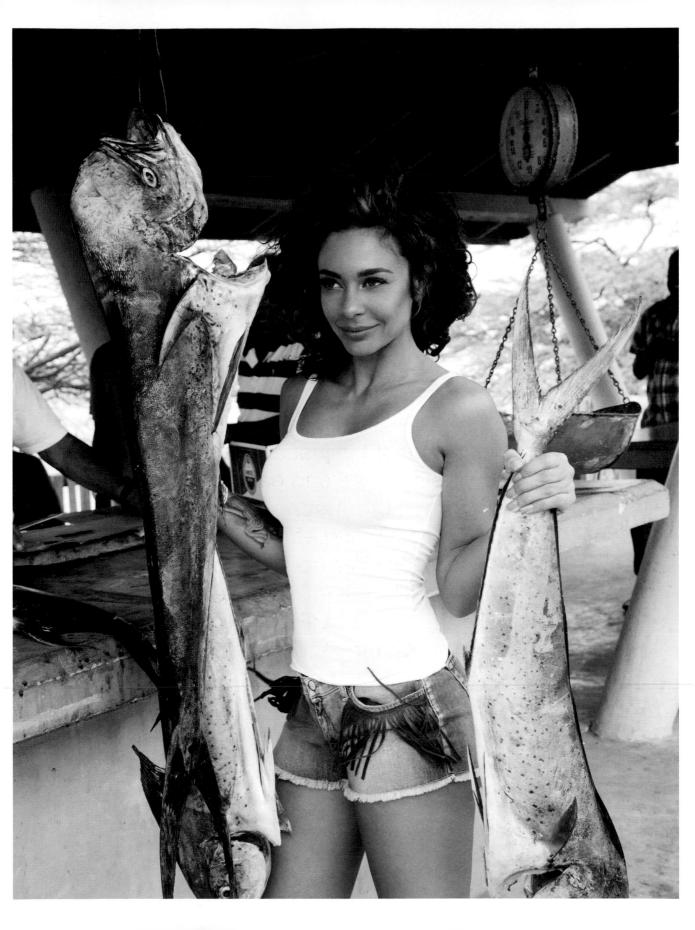

Not getting enough essential nutrients can really compromise your sports performance and get in the way of your goals, so a diet plan that is tailored to your personal needs is crucial. There is a lot of hype nowadays around superfoods and supplements promising miracles. These are all well and good, but getting the basics right is actually much more important, because that will provide the strong foundation your body needs. I will discuss this in more detail later, but what 'eating well' boils down to is simply eating fresh, healthy and unprocessed foods as much as possible. It really doesn't get any more complicated than this and, trust me, you will discover a whole new world by cutting out all those processed, refined foods. And the more you do so, the more you will see the benefits and actually enjoy the taste of a good healthy meal! You will find plenty of delicious recipes to inspire you later, in the Recipes chapter from page 166.

Basic nutrients

The right balance of carbohydrates, fats, proteins, vitamins and minerals will give you the energy you need, especially when training, but how much you need will actually depend on your gender, age, weight, and normal activity levels on any given day.

'WHAT WILL MAKE THE DIFFERENCE IS A HEALTHY, BALANCED DIET'

If you burn fewer calories than you take in, your body stores the excess, causing you to gain weight (described as a 'positive energy balance'). Conversely, if you burn more than you eat, your body starts using its reserves, causing you to lose weight (described as 'negative energy balance'). So having reached your target weight, the aim is to keep eating healthily and ensure your calorie intake matches the energy requirements of your body.

But if, aside from that, you also want to develop the perfect killer body, it is a little harder to get the balance right. This is why it is so important for you to decide on your personal goal. If it is building muscle, you will need a positive energy balance; if it is losing fat, a negative balance. But first things first: I will tell you a bit more about the three key nutrients – proteins, carbohydrates and fat, also known as 'macronutrients' or 'the macros'.

Macronutrients (macros)

Try googling 'If It Fits Your Macros' (IIFYM) – you'll get thousands of hits. So what are these macros? They are the proteins, carbohydrates and fats that give your body the energy it needs (how much will vary from person to person), while vitamins, minerals and trace elements, the so-called micronutrients, regulate body processes and functions. Our focus will be mainly on the macronutrients, which are especially important for building that perfect killer body.

Proteins

Proteins are primarily needed to build, maintain and repair muscle tissue; in other words, they are indispensable if you want to develop a muscular, toned look. The building blocks of proteins are 20 different amino acids, of which the non-essential ones are produced by the body itself, while the essential amino acids can only be obtained through diet. Animal protein is an excellent source, but no one food product will give you all the essential amino acids you need, so eating a variety of protein-rich foods is essential. Research shows that proteins are better than carbohydrates and fat for making you feel full, so they also have the benefit of reducing your appetite. Not that carbohydrates and fats don't matter – but more about these later.

SOURCES OF PROTEIN (1 GRAM OF PROTEIN = 4 CALORIES)

- Lean meat (chicken, turkey, beef)
- Fish
- Eggs
- Nuts, grains and pulses
- Quark

Carbohydrates

Carbohydrates are an important source of energy for your body, particularly the brain. The amount you need depends on things like gender and lifestyle. Your body converts carbohydrates into glucose, which is then quickly absorbed into the cells that can burn it to produce energy. But glucose can also be temporarily stored in your liver and muscle tissue (glycogen), which is useful for the occasional quick energy boost. While you often hear that too much carbohydrate will make you fat, there is no evidence to support that, although it is true that if you don't use up all the energy your body has produced, it will be stored and you will gain weight. Carbohydrates do contain a lot of calories, so watch out.

SOURCES OF CARBOHYDRATES (1 GRAM OF CARBOHYDRATE = 4 CALORIES)

- Potatoes
- Grain products such as bread, pasta and rice
- Fruit
- Pulses

'IF YOU DON'T USE UP ALL THE ENERGY YOUR BODY HAS PRODUCED, YOU WILL GAIN WEIGHT'

Fats

Fats often get the blame for weight gain. But make no mistake, they actually form a really important part of a healthy diet, providing energy and, moreover, essential vitamins A, D, E, as well as linoleic acid and alpha linolenic acid, two of the essential amino acids. It has recently been claimed that women especially can benefit from the positive effect of fats on hormones, heart and blood vessels.

Depending on their chemical structure, fats are either saturated or non-saturated. The amount of fat you need depends on whether you are male or female. But remember that fats give you more calories than either proteins or carbohydrates.

SOURCES OF FAT
(1 GRAM OF FAT = 8 CALORIES)

- Oily fish (eel, mackerel, herring, sardines, salmon)
- Nuts and seeds
- Avocado
- Oils
- Butter

TIPS

- Eat your greens! They contain a lot of fibre, vitamins and minerals, and have the added benefit of making you feel full.
- Drink plenty of water, at least 2 litres a day. Limit your intake of sugary drinks such as soft drinks and fruit juices.
- Choose whole grain products: wholewheat bread and pasta, brown rice etc.
- Cut out things you don't need that only add calories to your diet, such as snacks and alcohol.
- Do not buy any food you are not allowed to eat, because if it's there, you will.
- Get enough sleep: 7 to 9 hours is ideal. While you sleep, your body produces growth hormones, which promote muscle growth and the burning of fat reserves.

What makes a carbohydrate?

There is so much fuss about carbohydrates nowadays. For one, they are supposed to make you fat. And while some people will be convinced that 'it's the same as sugar', others will retort 'but you do actually need carbohydrates as well' and so on. That is why I wanted to dedicate a chapter to the carbohydrates because it's clear that some clarification is needed.

Simple versus complex

To start with, not all carbs are the same. It is tricky to differentiate between them without making it look very complicated, but if we look at their chemical structure we can distinguish between simple and complex carbohydrates, which gives us an idea of how fast the sugar is digested and absorbed. Examples of simple carbohydrates are fructose (fruit sugar), lactose (milk sugar) and sucrose ('ordinary' sugar). Complex carbohydrates, sometimes referred to as starch, are found in pulses, potatoes, rice and grain products.

The glycaemic index

The World Health Organisation and the Food and Agriculture Organisation have ranked foods according to their 'glycaemic index', or GI-value. This index ranges from 0 to 100, looking at the speed at which blood sugar levels rise after eating different kinds of foods. High GI foods are digested and absorbed at a much faster rate, resulting in rapid fluctuations in blood sugar levels. This is in contrast with low-GI foods, which are digested and absorbed more slowly and cause a slower rise in blood sugar levels.

Ever wondered how you can tell the difference between fast and slow carbs? Well, the GI will give you a clue. Slow-carb foods often have a low GI-value and the lower the GI the better they are for your health. This is because the instant boost of energy you get from high-GI products (fast carbohydrates) will be quickly followed by a dip, making you feel tired, drained and peckish again.

But are slow carbohydrates necessarily better than fast carbohydrates for developing your physique? The answer is no. One study (that compared products similar both in terms of the amount of energy they provided and their balance of macronutrients but with varying

'ENERGY IS MEASURED IN CALORIES, NOT CARBOHYDRATES'

GI-values) concluded that the effect of these products on muscle mass or fat loss was no different.

In other words, sugars are sugars, whether you eat a Snickers bar or a bowl of rice with the equivalent amount of carbohydrates. But although it will make no difference to your diet, it will of course have an impact on your health.

Sports performance

The GI-value of the food you eat before training does not have a bearing on your endurance, either; the idea that 'you need carbohydrates for energy' is a myth. Energy is actually measured in calories, not carbohydrates. So when it comes to developing physique, it makes no difference whether the carbohydrates are simple or complex, or whether their GI is high or low. What matters is the total carbohydrate count in your diet, because carbohydrates contain calories.

A note of caution here: don't take this as a cue for eating all the sweets and other carbohydrate-rich foods you like without giving it a second thought. There is a difference between the 'empty' calories in sugar, for instance, and the calories you get from eating a sweet potato. The sweet potato may have the same amount of sugar but also contains other micronutrients that are good for you, which makes it far more beneficial.

Sugar

The other drawback of sugar is that it scores very low on the so-called 'satiety index', so it doesn't fill you up. Worse, adding sugar to your meals can actually make you eat more, because it tastes good. But does that necessarily make sugar the 'forbidden fruit'? Are the calories in sugar 'worse' than the calories in carbohydrates? This has also been extensively researched, and the results show that as long as your total calorie intake remains the same, you can substitute the complex carbohydrates (low GI) with sugar without any detrimental effect – at least in terms of the impact on your physique.

But again, eating a chocolate bar will not fill you up the way a sweet potato does, even though the calorie intake is actually the same. So after that bar of chocolate, it is more than likely you will want to eat something else, and that will make you go over your daily calorie limit. The lesson here is that it's fine to eat the occasional chocolate treat, as long as you eat it instead of your bowl of rice or sweet potato – if it 'fits your macros', you can eat anything!

My personal food favourites

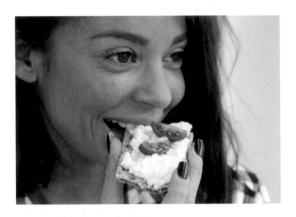

Cottage cheese

This is one of my favourites. Cottage cheese is rich in protein and only contains 3.9% fat, and is delicious with all sorts of foods. Try putting it on a light crispy cracker with a slice of cooked chicken breast and a tomato or with a dash of cinnamon and a drop of honey for a sweet evening treat. I also really like it with just a few apple slices.

Coffee

Coffee not only tastes great, but if you drink it in moderation it can even be beneficial. It contains antioxidants and speeds up your metabolism, meaning you burn more calories even when resting. I drink about 3 cups a day and although I much prefer to have it with milk, this cancels out its positive effects, so I restrict myself to only one cup with skimmed milk.

I start the day with a glass of water and a cup of black coffee and then go off to do my training. I don't find it hard to train on an empty stomach, because the coffee gives me the energy I need, and I actually prefer it. Coffee really keeps me going when I am doing IF (Intermittent Fasting, see page 55). It stills your hunger, which is very convenient if you are fasting for at least part of the day, or even just dieting. It is so nice not to feel those hunger pangs. Black coffee will help you stick to your diet more easily and, moreover, it contains no calories!

But the list of advantages doesn't end there. Caffeine triggers several hormones, adrenaline, dopamine and cortisol, and all three have the same effect, which is to effectively put your body in 'fight or flight' mode – as when you are under stress. Your body responds by rapidly converting the amino acids in your muscles and the glycogen in your liver into glucose in the blood. Burning that glucose will produce a lot of energy, giving a nice little boost to your sports performance!

A note of caution, though: drinking coffee will not necessarily help you achieve all your goals – cortisol can actually have an adverse effect if you are trying to build muscle, for example.

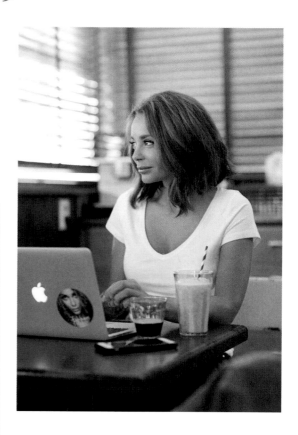

Green coffee

Most of us associate coffee with black roasted beans, but there is actually such a thing as green coffee. Green coffee beans have not been burnt or roasted, and so retain more of the antioxidants. Green coffee allegedly speeds up your metabolism even more than normal coffee.

DRAWBACKS OF COFFEE

Coffee does have a dark side. The obvious disadvantages are:

- The sugar, milk or cream you add to it also adds calories.
- Drinking too much coffee gives you a surplus of glucose, which is converted into sugars and fats.
- Coffee raises blood sugar levels, which stimulates the production of adrenaline.
- Drinking too much will make you feel tired and disturb your sleep, which hampers weight loss.

REDUCE CELLULITE WITH A COFFEE SCRUB

It's not exactly the best-kept beauty secret that scrubbing removes dead skin cells and stimulates circulation. Poor skin circulation is one of the causes of cellulite, so scrubbing your skin is an effective way to reduce it. I scrub myself once a week with the grounds from my coffee machine, but if you don't have one, why not get one of those old fashioned little coffee pots? Or there are many other products out there to buy if you'd prefer. Not only does a coffee scrub soften the skin, but the caffeine also reduces fluid retention and dilates the blood vessels, thereby stimulating the blood flow in the skin. The antioxidants in coffee also remove toxins, plus a coffee scrub supposedly helps you burn fat faster.

Cellulite

Cellulite is probably the thing that upsets me the most when I look at my body, and if the volume of messages I get about the subject (a third of the total) are anything to go by, it seems I share this with quite a lot of women. Pleased as I am with my hourglass figure, unfortunately this makes me relatively more prone to cellulite than someone with, say, an apple-shaped body. The fat tends to go straight to my buttocks and legs, and those horrible dimples are the tell-tale signs.

My cellulite got really bad during my 2 pregnancies, because of all the oestrogen my body was producing. Fortunately much of it disappeared afterwards, but it reared its ugly head again after I took part in *Expedition Robinson* and also during my training for the New York marathon. That was because my body was producing too many stress hormones, while at the same time I was also eating a lot of soy products, which stimulate the production of oestrogen.

'I THINK I HAVE TRIED PRETTY MUCH EVERY TREATMENT GOING OVER THE YEARS'

But I finally have it under contol. Not that I am completely free of the problem, but I can live with the amount I have. I think I have tried pretty much every treatment going over the years, only to conclude that sadly, nothing really works. So be wary of miracle cures, all those creams, special treatments or training offered by companies that often have only one motive: profit. Just make sure you know what you are signing up for.

Here are some of the different treatments I have tried . . .

ENDERMOLOGY (GYMNASTICS ON THE SKIN)

A mechanical massage therapy, this didn't work at all for me. But some people seem to get positive results, if only temporarily.

SHOCKWAVE THERAPY

Very painful and costly, but the three treatments per week I had did actually work. The results were visible after about ten treatments, though the dimples returned as soon as I stopped. Once, in America, I had little injections into each and every dimple, supposedly to dissolve the fat and make them disappear. Stupidly, I did it just before a photoshoot. I ended up with 200 bruises on my legs, and all the dimples still there.

ALGAE WRAPS

The least costly treatment, and the advice is to only have it done twice. You will look slimmer after the treatment, and may actually go down a dress size, but that is only because of the loss of fluids. So make the most of your new svelte look, because it will only last one evening.

CONNECTIVE TISSUE MASSAGE

As long as you eat well, are physically active and drink plenty of water, it is not a bad idea to have a connective tissue massage about once a week. It is very painful, but it does help rid your body of toxins.

What is cellulite?

Cellulite is a condition in which subcutaneous fat causes dimpling of the skin, giving it the appearance and feel of orange peel – hence it is commonly referred to as 'orange peel skin'. But let's be clear: cellulite is not to be confused with cellulitis, which is a bacterial infection of the subcutaneous connective tissue that often causes redness, swelling and fever. Cellulite, on the other hand, is not an infection, but the result of fatty deposits within the underlying connective tissue of the skin.

Causes

If you have cellulite, you are not alone, so don't feel embarrassed about it. Some 90% of all women admit to having it, though some worse than others. Oestrogen, the female hormone, can have a particularly marked effect on the skin during puberty, pregnancy and the menopause. Smoking is also bad for cellulite, so it's best not to, or at least to cut down.

Cellulite has a number of different causes, including:

- Stagnation of blood flow and lymphatic congestion with fluid retention. Toxins are then trapped in the body and nestle between the fat cells

- Fat cells clogging up and swelling together
- Connective tissue adhesions
- Loss of skin elasticity
- Genetic predisposition
- Liver problems, for example due to alcohol
- Poor sleeping patterns
- Medical causes or medication

You may find that not all of these apply to you: cellulite can be the result of just a few of these problems.

Diet and stress

Stress is another cause of cellulite. It has a detrimental effect on the skin because it disturbs the processing of fats and the body's hormonal balance. It also affects your breathing, reducing the amount of oxygen you take in, which also impacts on your metabolism and sleeping patterns. And if you don't sleep well, your body doesn't get the rest it needs to recuperate and restore.

Hormones

Hormones are often the main culprit, especially when there is an imbalance between oestrogen and testosterone levels, as relatively high oestrogen often causes cellulite. Using the pill also increases your chances of getting it.

Yo-yo effect

Cellulite is also caused by weight cycling, otherwise known as the yo-yo effect, as your skin will gradually lose elasticity. Cellulite consists of fat cells, which grow when you gain weight, making the cellulite more pronounced. As you gain weight, the dimples will get deeper, but when you shed the excess weight again, they will not reduce back to the size they were.

Cellulite has three levels: at the lowest level it is only discernible when you actually squeeze the skin or tense your muscles; at the medium level it is slightly visible, though more so when you tense your muscles, while at the highest level it is very pronounced, and always clearly visible.

Treatment

Remember, all types of cellulite are very hard to reduce. If it's only minor, you may be able to treat it but if the metabolism of your skin is disturbed, it will require specialist treatment by a beautician, masseur and/or physiotherapist. A combination of power- and cardio-training may help reduce it, as will cutting back on alcohol and minimising stress. You could also consider a break from taking the pill, to control your hormones. Obviously, healthy eating and ensuring your weight remains stable are also key.

Sports and exercise

Building muscle mass underneath the cellulite will visibly reduce it, as the skin will become more taut. In any case, exercising will improve circulation and can reduce fatty deposits as well. If you combine a healthy lifestyle and exercise with a sensible, balanced diet, you are much less likely to get cellulite, and to reduce it, you should moderate your intake of:

- Dairy
- Coffee (no more than three cups a day)
- Sugar
- Soy
- Chocolate
- Pastries
- Soft drinks

Lastly, eat as many hard green vegetables as you can, take DIM tablets (after getting appropriate medical advice), which help reduce oestrogen dominance, and use your coffee grounds to give yourself a really good scrub once a week!

How to stick to your diet

How can you ensure that you never stray from your healthy eating habits? Well, it's all in the preparation. Get everything you need when you go grocery shopping, and take your own food wherever you go. If you always take your own food to work, school or a function, chances are you will be able to resist temptation. This is why the first 12 weeks of #MKBM only include lunch recipes that are easy for you to take with you.

A few more tips:

- Do your food shop once a week using the shopping list in this book, and don't be tempted to put anything else in your trolley.
- Prepare the salads for lunch a day ahead, and keep them in the fridge to save time in the morning.
- Always prepare meals a day or even 2 days ahead if you are busy.
- Make sure you don't buy anything you don't really need.

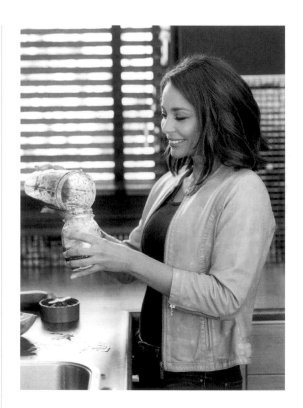

Eating on holiday

Whenever I go away, I prefer to rent a house, to avoid being dependent on restaurants. While I really enjoy going out to dinner, I often can't help eating just that little bit too much and find it particularly hard to resist the desserts afterwards. Not that it's bad to have something sweet now and again, certainly not on holiday, but if you do it every day . . . All too often, you pile the pounds back on during your break and all your efforts go to waste in the space of a few weeks.

So here are my tips for making sure your killer body survives the holidays:

- Try to rent an apartment rather than staying in a hotel, so that you can cook your own food.
- If you do book a hotel or resort, check they have a gym. If they don't, chances are that you will not keep up your exercise regime.
- The food in restaurants tends to be a little more fatty than what you'd prepare at home, so try eating fewer carbohydrates to compensate.
- Try to have a protein-rich breakfast and stay well away from the croissants and muffins. Starting the day with all that sugar only makes your body want more throughout the rest of the day.
- Record your calorie intake with an app, to help you keep track of what you eat.
- Don't drink too much alcohol. Choose a special day to drink and don't be persuaded that every day is a special day.
- I love to go hiking when I am on holiday, and start out with an empty stomach – apart from a cup of black espresso, which helps burn fat. And then I head for the hills!

How can I maintain my weight?

How can you maintain your weight after you've finished the plan? As I mentioned earlier, it boils down to the right diet, which will make your training more effective to help you reach your goal. If you want to build muscle and tone your body as well, the quantity and the quality of what you eat and drink will be crucial. So in this chapter I will explain how you can devise your own personal diet plan that is perfect for what you want to achieve. Everyone is different, which is why the perfect diet plan will vary from person to person, depending on your gender, age, daily activities and body fat percentage.

Quantity relates to the macronutrient ratios in your diet (see page 33), while quality is about getting all the nutrients you need from a range of fresh products. In a nutshell: make sure that you eat the right amount of proteins, carbohydrates and fats to attain your particular goal, and get the nutrition you need from a variety of fresh, unprocessed foods.

TIP

Don't lose sight of your goal, and just go for it! Do everything you can to stick to your diet, for example taking your own food wherever you go (work, function, a birthday or party) to avoid the temptation of popping into the canteen or having just a little bit of that birthday cake. Have you already succumbed or think you might? Then plan to go training on that day or the day after so that you can at least burn off the extra calories.

Four steps

Devising your own diet plan begins with calculating your personal daily calorie needs. This will tell you how much of the macronutrients (proteins, carbohydrates and fats) you should incorporate into your diet to build muscle. Follow these 4 steps:

- Define your goal: what do you want to achieve?
- Calculate your energy needs.
- Devise your own personal diet plan: what is suitable for your body?
- Evaluate: has your plan had the desired effect?

'IT IS PHYSICALLY IMPOSSIBLE TO BURN FAT AND BUILD MUSCLE AT THE SAME TIME'

1 Define your goal

The first step is to decide exactly what it is you want to achieve, and set yourself a time frame. Your goals should be realistic – I can't say this often enough: if they're not, you'll only end up feeling disappointed and demoralised. So it's basically a choice between these two options:

- You want to lose fat without losing muscle
- You want to build muscle without gaining fat

Is it even possible to burn fat and build muscle at the same time? The fact is, you need a negative energy balance (when your body uses up energy reserves) to lose weight, but a positive energy balance (when your body stores energy) to build muscle. Or, to put it differently, losing weight is a catabolic process (breaking down), while building muscle (and so gaining weight) is anabolic. The answer lies in a combination of power- and cardio-training (HIIT or High Intensity Interval Training) that will enable you to build muscle and simultaneously burn a lot of calories, as muscle burns more calories than fat does. So it is better to do cardio-training in combination with other exercise.

Taking that into consideration, a clear, realistic goal for a two-month training period might be for example to lose 4% of your body fat without losing any muscle.

Do remember that the closer you get to your target, the harder it will get. You will find that the first 2% are the quickest and easiest to lose, but the last 2% may seem a real struggle and take more time. And to make it worse, as you lose weight, you will need fewer calories, so your diet should be adapted accordingly. That's if you want to keep losing weight, of course.

2 Calculate your energy needs

The key question is: how much protein, carbohydrates and fat do you need to incorporate into your diet? Well, this depends on your body fat percentage, and you can actually measure this using a device called a skinfold caliper. It's probably best to get the first measurement done by a qualified professional either at the gym or a dietician's practice, so you start with the right baseline figure. If you then decide you want to monitor your own progress, you can buy a decent caliper for around £6.

The next thing you need to know is your 'maintenance calorie intake' – that is the amount of calories you need to maintain your current body weight. If you take in fewer (also referred to as 'cutting', see page 86), your body fat will be reduced; if you take in more (known as 'bulking', see page 82), you will gain muscle. The table below tells you how you can calculate your maintenance calories: simply multiply your weight by the relevant figure, depending on your body type (see page 22).

ECTOMORPH	weight × 44
MESOMOPH	weight × 33
ENDOMORPH	weight × 26

TIP

If you want to lose weight a bit more quickly, one option is not to compensate for the extra calories you have burned by training. For example: your maintenance intake is 1500 calories a day, but you consume only 1300 because you are trying to lose weight. You train for 1 hour 3 times a week, which burns 200 calories each time. So you could allow yourself an additional 200 calories on those days and still lose weight, because of the exercise. But if you stick to the 1300 calories a day limit, even on the days you have exercised, you will obviously lose weight faster.

3 Create your diet plan

When you create your own diet plan, you should know the daily calorie intake you are aiming for, and the relative proportions of macronutrients that will be required to achieve it. The average workout will derive 40% of the required calories from proteins, 30% from carbs, and 30% from fats.

Here is a list of foods grouped by macronutrient:

PROTEINS
- Lean meat (chicken, turkey, beef)
- Fish
- Eggs
- Nuts, grains, pulses
- Quark

CARBOHYDRATES

Slow carbs
(These are absorbed more slowly so, it takes longer for the starch to be converted into glucose)
- Whole grain pasta/ bread
- Brown rice
- Vegetables
- Quinoa
- Oats

Fast carbs
(These raise the blood sugar levels quickly but only for a short time, making you more hungry and tired afterwards)
- Fruit

FATS
- Oily fish (eel, mackerel, herring, sardines, salmon)
- Avocado
- Seeds
- Peanut butter
- Nuts

4 Evaluate your diet plan

Don't expect your first plan to be spot on straight away. You will probably need to evaluate it about every four weeks, and perhaps make a few adjustments to make sure it is appropriate for your body. How effective it is will also depend on your metabolism, which can change over time – certainly for women, as we know all too well. Don't make any drastic changes though, and introduce any adjustments gradually. If needs be, take advice from a qualified professional at the gym or consult a dietician.

Remember also that as you lose weight you will need fewer calories, so you should eat less and less if you want to keep losing weight. If you feel that you are not getting the results you want, you may need to look at the macro ratios again. The ones I have given you are just guidelines; it really all depends on how your body responds. As for me, I know I do really well as long as I keep my carbs at 20%, but you may be one of those people who needs to keep their fats at 20%.

Healthy products that can hamper your success

This will probably sound familiar: you spend an evening on the sofa, watching a film, and you feel a little peckish. Aha, you think, I'll go for some nuts rather than crisps, because they're healthier, right?

The answer is no. I'm afraid not. Yes, nuts do have a lot of good nutrients, but they are also high in calories, which you should be watching if you are trying to lose weight; using up more energy than you consume, remember? So those healthy, 'innocent' snacks can really throw a spanner in the works!

Avocado is another typical example: we put it on a cracker, in a salad and in the guacamole. It just keeps popping up in our diet and is becoming ever more popular. But although this healthy fruit does contain the right fats and important nutrients, it also has a lot of calories. No need to cross it off the shopping list altogether, but do take care that you don't have too many of them: too much of a good thing can actually ruin your chances of getting a killer body.

And that brings me to yet another popular phenomenon: superfoods. Are you one of those people who swears by throwing gojiberries, mulberries and the like into your yogurt by the handful every morning?

You must have guessed what I am about to tell you. Yes, they are healthy – if eaten in large quantities, which also means a lot of calories. I hate to disappoint you, but there are simply no miracle substances that will speed up the process of developing your killer body. Just make sure you get your 5 a day, that's healthy enough.

Would you like to know more about what works and what doesn't, and even get a diet plan tailormade especially for you? Then register your details on my website: www.mykillerbodymotivation.com.

Eat to lose fat! Refeed!

Once you have followed the #MKBM diet for 12 weeks and lost enough weight, I would strongly advise you not to go back to your old eating habits, but to carry on with the diet as you did in Phase 1. It will be absolutely fine to plan a cheat meal once a week as well, though of course you could also choose to try and lose more weight, or build more dry muscle and lower your body fat percentage a little more. Once your body fat drops below 14%, you can carry on with the Phase 3 diet, and have a refeed day once a week. I often get asked about refeeds via my website and social media, and have on previous occasions quipped about my refeeding habits involving vodka, but obviously that is just a joke and really not a good idea.

So all jokes aside: I will explain the purpose of a refeed and how you should go about it. If you are really keen to try it, there is a refeed plan later in this book which you can follow during the final phase of the weight loss diet. By that stage, your body fat should have dropped to a level where you actually need to refeed once a week anyway, which is great, as it is simply a way of losing more fat – how bad can that be?

The final phase of the 12-week diet includes a refeed every Sunday, by the end of which you should have reached your target weight – if you haven't, just carry on with the last phase of the diet for a few more weeks. The best way to maintain your ideal weight will then be to go back to the Phase 1 diet. If your body fat percentage is below normal (around 25% for a woman and 22% for a man), you will need to refeed every week, but if it's above that level, you won't – though you can still incorporate a weekly cheat meal if you like.

Refeeding is a way of countering the effect of two hormones, leptin and ghrelin, which are responsible for regulating your appetite and fat burning. Ghrelin is produced in the stomach (the fundus, the upper part of the stomach) and it increases before meals, making you feel hungry, then drops after you have eaten.

Ghrelin works in tandem with leptin, which sends a signal to the brain that you are full once you have eaten enough to store sufficient energy in your fat cells (the fat cells release the leptin). But when you eat less (to lose weight), you consequently burn more of those fat cells, and the reduced leptin levels make your body think that you are not yet full and still need to eat more. The natural response is to then ration the use of energy from fat cells and this is where the refeed comes in: it counters this rationing effect.

Refeed day

You lose weight by using more energy than you consume. Refeeding is a way of redressing the balance by eating the amount of calories you would normally need to maintain your body weight (not gaining or losing any weight, as explained in the chapter about calculating your calorie needs), or perhaps eating a little more.

It seems counter-intuitive to think that when you refeed, you are in fact eating to lose more weight. But when you take in fewer calories than you really need, the leptin and ghrelin slow your metabolism down – it is your body's natural response, that survival instinct from our hunter-gatherer days when food was often a little harder to come by. Useful back then, but not when you are actually trying to lose weight.

'REFEEDING IS A WAY OF COUNTERING THE EFFECT OF TWO HORMONES, LEPTIN AND GHRELIN'

'REFEEDING EFFECTIVELY MEANS A LITTLE REPROGRAMMING OF YOUR BODY'

Refeeding is really just a way of fooling your body to prevent this natural reaction. It works by bringing your leptin levels back up so that your metabolism increases, your hunger pangs wane, and all goes back to normal. Effectively just a little reprogramming of your body so that it's happy to believe that 'energy levels are up, crisis is over – let's get back to work and burn those calories.'

There is a big 'but', however: don't be tricked into thinking you can just eat anything you like; it really doesn't work like that. I would certainly steer clear of all fats, and choose mainly foods that are high in complex carbs, such as rice, potatoes and vegetables, which have a much bigger impact on your leptin levels.

There are a few other good reasons for refeeding I should mention here. When you lose weight, it causes stress to your body (hence the survival mode) which releases cortisol, the stress hormone responsible for breaking down muscle. As refeeding increases your leptin levels, it also lowers the cortisol, protecting your muscle tissue. Finally, an ongoing calorie deficit can make you more prone to illness, so refeeding will effectively give your immune system a boost – and of course a day of being allowed to eat a bit more is likely to boost your morale as well!

Guidelines

You should follow these guidelines when you are planning a refeed:

- Eat around 500 calories above your maintenance level.
- Plan to have your refeed day before a training day where you focus on the large muscle groups, to give you more energy for that training.
- Eat complex carbohydrates and steer clear of fats. Sweet potatoes, rice, pasta and lots of vegetables are good.
- Restrict proteins to one gram per kilogram of body weight.
- Keep products with high fructose (sugar) content to a minimum.

How often you should refeed depends on your gender and body fat percentage:

WOMEN

> 30% FAT	no refeed required
25–30% FAT	1 × every 2 weeks
16–25% FAT	1 × every week
< 16% FAT	2 × every week

MEN

> 20% FAT	no refeed required
15–20% FAT	1 × every 2 weeks
12–15% FAT	1 × every week
< 12% FAT	2 × every week

'REFEEDING IS LIKELY TO BOOST YOUR MORALE AS WELL'

Intermittent Fasting

I am a big fan of Intermittent Fasting (IF), which means not eating or drinking any calories for 16–20 hours on a particular day and then making up for the 'lost' calories for that day within the remaining hours.

It basically forces your body to start using up fat reserves. A lot of people think you should eat every two hours to keep your metabolism high, but that is not true: your body only starts to store fat if you stop eating for more than 60 hours, or when your body fat percentage is very low.

IF can be done during #MKBM, in the first instance to lose fat and then to build dry muscle mass (muscle without fat). Once you have reached those goals, you can still carry on fasting intermittently now and again to keep your body fat low.

There are different methods of IF, and many online sources available if you want to find out more about IF and losing weight, as I have kept the information here to a minimum.

The essential things to know about IF is that you can follow an IF programme for as long as you like, but it is advisable to take a break from it after 12 weeks, for two weeks, during which you eat the amount of calories you normally would to maintain your body weight (see page 46). You can then start another 12-week stint. Plan to fast for about 16–20 hours each day – it doesn't really matter what part of the day – and then make up for the lost calories during the remaining 4–8 hours.

'IT DOESN'T REALLY MATTER WHAT PART OF THE DAY YOU CHOOSE TO FAST'

It might seem impossible to go without anything that contains calories for such a big part of the day, but believe me, it is not as hard as it sounds. I have found the easiest way is to skip breakfast and just eat my first meal a bit later in the day.

Don't forget that the hours you sleep also count as IF hours, so those are in the bag already! And then 4–8 hours after waking (depending on your preference and experience of IF), you can enjoy eating and drinking all your calories for the day within the next 4–8 hours. Most people who do IF plan to have their meals between midday and 8 p.m. Not really that difficult, is it?

But you can be as flexible as you like, of course, and choose a different part of the day each time – plan it around a busy day at work, a hefty training session or a wild party you're looking forward to.

Result

But the key question is of course: why bother? Well, if you consider that IF will help you lose around 500–750 grams of fat per week, that should convince you. The exact amount will of course depend on how high your body fat percentage is – the more fat, the faster it burns to begin with. Once that starts to drop, your weight loss will slow down as well – as it should, because if you lose weight too fast, your metabolism slows and your body then starts to break down muscle to produce energy.

Speaking of losing weight, a few more advantages of IF:

- It makes your body produce more growth hormones, which stimulate the burning of fat reserves, help in the building and repair of muscle and improve your metabolism.
- It increases your insulin sensitivity. Insulin is a hormone that is responsible for transporting carbohydrates to all the cells in the body. Increased sensitivity makes the carbs go to your muscle rather than the fat cells.
- It makes your body produce more noradrenaline, a hormone that stimulates your metabolism and makes you more alert and productive.

IF has other health-related advantages:

- It improves your cardiovascular system
- It reduces risk of heart disease
- It reduces stress
- It lengthens your lifespan

In short, there's a lot to gain without too much effort, planning or preparation involved!

No wonder I am such a big IF enthusiast, as I'm sure you will be too, once you start. And think of this: it's another step closer to your killer body!

Healthy, humanely produced meat

As I mentioned earlier, hormones play a big part in weight and physical development. But what many people don't realise is that our meat all too often contains added hormones (for example growth hormones) and other additives such as antibiotics, which have been injected into the animals. This obviously is not healthy at the best of times, and it worsens the problem of our antibiotics resistance as well. It is one of the reasons I increasingly opt for a vegetarian diet, and make up for the lost proteins with BCAA supplements and protein shakes. When I do eat meat, I buy it online from an organic source.

Chicken

Much of the chicken we eat is full of antibiotics, as the vast majority of chicken farmers (including organic ones!) cannot afford to work without them because of the ESBL (extended-spectrum beta-lactamases) enzymes and salmonella bacteria. These ESBL enzymes are especially dangerous as they make bacteria resistant to antibiotics. This is why much of the antibiotic treatment given to chickens is preventative.

However, this antibiotics resistance will be passed on to us if we eat a lot of chicken. And to make matters worse, the chickens are often given growth hormones as well, to turn them into oversized, 2-kilo birds within a mere six weeks! This cannot be right for either the chicken or ourselves. It may be harder to find, but if you can buy completely organic, free-range chicken, fed on a natural diet that ensures they have not been subjected to antibiotic and growth hormone treatment, all the better.

Beef

You may be able to find 'grass-fed' organic beef either in the shops or online, produced from cows that have been allowed to graze freely and that have eaten only grass, without any antibiotics or special power feeds to supplement their diet. The problem with these animal feeds is that alongside grains they also contains soy, which, as I mentioned earlier, stimulates the production of oestrogen, the hormone responsible for fat on the hips and thighs, as well as cellulite (only if you are a woman, of course).

The grains and soy have another hidden cost: the destruction of rainforests, which is yet another good reason not to buy anything but grass-fed. Grass is far better for the cows, for the environment and ultimately for ourselves. Grass-fed organic beef contains more omega 3 fatty acids, CLA (Conjugated Linoleic Acid, see page 60) and vitamins A and E. And believe me, once you have tasted it, you will never look back.

Pork

Similarly, organic, free-range pork is raised humanely and is of a much better quality and taste, owing to the fact that the pigs have been reared outdoors on a natural diet that includes grass, herbs and mustard seeds as well as beet, wheat, barley, maize, rapeseed and sunflower meal, beet pulp and molasses. In other words, richly varied. Moreover, they are only treated with antibiotics if it is really necessary, never preventatively.

BCAA and other food supplements

BCAA stands for Branched Chain Amino Acid. Amino acids are the building blocks of proteins. Your body breaks down proteins to produce its own amino acids, which it then distributes to different parts of your body where they are needed to repair, build and strengthen tissue, including muscle.

There are essential and non-essential amino acids. While the non-essential amino acids are produced by your own body, you can only obtain the essential ones through your diet (particularly from eating dairy, eggs, legumes and meat). Around 35–40% of BCAA's essential amino acids are derived from food, and they form 14–18% of all amino acids in muscle protein. So they are important!

But why take BCAA supplements if you can get these amino acids through eating the right foods, anyway? The answer is that, as with all other supplements, they are not intended as a replacment for food but as an additional source of nutrients – just make sure you get enough of them.

Besides, BCAA does actually differ from the amino acids you get from food, as the latter require some 'processing' in the liver before they can be used – and they are used only if they are needed for energy. BCAA, on the other hand, goes straight to the muscles, and if it's not needed for fuel (because there are already sufficient fats and carbohydrates available), it sets to work on building and repairing muscle.

'PEOPLE WHO WORK OUT A LOT PROBABLY NEED TO TOP UP THE AMINO ACIDS THEY GET FROM THEIR FOOD'

Research has also shown that BCAA lowers the cortisol levels (the stress hormone) in your body. Sports causes stress to the body, and cortisol breaks down muscle, but BCAA counters this effect. And in any case, people who work out a lot probably need to top up the amino acids they get from their food, and you should count yourself among them if you are training for a killer body!

Other supplements I use are fish oil and CLA tablets, as well as multivitamins and vitamin D during the winter months. A little more information about these follows below.

Fish oil

Fish oil supplies essential fatty acids (omega 3 fatty acids EPA and DHA) which we often don't get in sufficient quantities through our diet. If you don't eat oily fish at least twice a week, it might be a good idea to take one or two fish oil capsules a day. A few more advantages:

- Fish oil reduces fat storage: it ensures that our body cells absorb insulin more easily.
- Improves your mood by increasing serotonin levels.
- EPA helps to keep joints supple.
- Improves concentration by stimulating blood supply to the brain.

CLA

Another essential amino acid is omega 6, found in CLA tablets. They are good for reducing fat and building muscle as CLA helps reduce fat storage, encourages muscle gain, protects the muscle tissue and improves metabolism.

Multivitamins and vitamin D

If you are no big fan of fruit, it is advisable to take some multivitamins with your first meal of the day; I only do this during the winter months, because your resistance can be a bit lower then. Multivitamins contain minerals and vitamins that are often not present in sufficient quantities in the average diet, and if you are very active (for example during #MKBM) your body will need more of these nutrients. You can obviously adjust your diet to increase your intake, but a little extra always helps.

I also take some vitamin D, which is very important for strong bones and teeth. Your body can actually produce it in sufficient quantities if you are exposed to enough sunlight, but if not, or during the winter months, many people can really benefit from taking extra vitamin D. Foods such as oily fish, meat and eggs have naturally high levels of vitamin D, but it is also added to other products like margarine.

Proteins for vegetarians

Proteins derived from food are digested and broken down into amino acids (as explained in the previous chapter). Your body needs 20 different ones: 9 essential (which you get from food) and 11 non-essential (which your body itself produces). Your body can't produce the essential amino acids.

Your body also needs all the essential amino acids in the right proportions for them to be converted into 'complete proteins'. But as a vegetarian, you will find it more difficult to get all these amino acids through your diet, because meat is a main source. However, by cleverly combining eggs, cheese, yogurt, quark and milk with other foods, you should be OK. A few examples:

- Pea soup with wholewheat or brown bread
- Brown rice with chickpeas
- Bread and egg
- Rice and brown (pinto) beans
- Rice with taho, tofu, a vegetarian burger or Quorn
- Lentils with rice
- Rice with cashew nuts and/or sesame seeds
- Chickpeas and couscous
- Nut loaf
- Mushrooms with brown rice
- Mushroom soup with peas and rye bread

Omega 3

Oily fish (herring, salmon, mackerel and sardines) is the most important source of omega 3 fatty acids, the healthy fats we cannot do without. We need them to produce hormones and to nourish our brains, improve our mood, behaviour and mental agility. Our metabolism increases, fat storage is reduced and infections are inhibited. These fatty acids improve the immune system and are beneficial for the cardiovascular system. This means that eating oily fish really is a must at least 2 or 3 times a week. If you don't, make sure you take fish oil supplements.

Shellfish

Shellfish is an important source of iodine, zinc and selenium. You need iodine and selenium for your thyroid gland, which in turn promotes good metabolism and temperature regulation.

Oestrogen dominance

The influence of some hormones on your body weight and development have already been mentioned. As a mother of two I am well aware that pregnancy hormones can really bring about big changes in your body, including oestrogen dominance, which can cause a lot of bother.

If it is only temporary – as during pregnancy – all you can do is ride out the storm, knowing it will pass, and perhaps follow the advice generally given for oestrogen dominance, which can be helpful. It is a subject close to my heart as women who suffer with it are much more prone to cellulite and storing fat on the hips and thighs. All I can say is don't lose hope, there are ways of dealing with it!

Oestrogen, the female sex hormone, has a very important role to play in fertility, good health and preventing infections. It is only when it is too high in relation to other hormones such as testosterone and progesterone, a condition referred to as oestrogen dominance, that it can cause trouble. There can be quite a few reasons for this imbalance, which I will not delve into here, but pregnancy certainly is one of them. The symptoms include:

- Mood swings
- Swollen and sometimes painful breasts
- Fluid retention
- Fat storage, especially on the hips and thighs
- Weight gain
- Feelings of depression and irritability
- Fatigue
- Headaches or migraines
- Candida (yeast infection)
- Acne (pimples)
- Magnesium deficiency
- Zinc deficiency
- Fibroids in the uterus

Some of these symptoms go hand in hand with pregnancy, so it can be hard to tell what's causing them. If in any doubt, consult a qualified professional.

Preventing or reducing oestrogen dominance

A healthy diet and lifestyle are the best remedies for oestrogen dominance and in fact, the two prerequisites for a healthy hormone balance. So the general advice is to eat well and take regular exercise. Some vegetables are also particularly beneficial as they contain a substance called diindolylmethane (DIM), which supports a healthy oestrogen metabolism which helps your hormone balance. DIM occurs naturally in the following vegetables, so make sure you incorporate plenty of these into your daily diet:

· Cauliflower
· Kale
· Broccoli
· Radishes
· Red cabbage
· Rocket
· Sprouts
· Cress
· White cabbage

It's always best to eat fresh and preferably organic vegetables as much as you can, but you can also juice them for a yummy DIM-packed smoothie or juice. If you are stretched for time or don't fancy getting your juicer out, DIM-tablets are a very good alternative as a quick, effective way to tackle oestrogen dominance. The best ones on the market are those with 'high bioavailability', as these are absorbed more easily. You can buy DIM supplements in health food shops or online.

How can I fit it all in?

People often post comments like, 'Well, I would look like that if I didn't have to work' or 'I'd kill for a body like yours' or 'How on earth do you find the time?' Often they simply cannot imagine how I manage to cram so much in and yet find the time to be a good mum. But that's nonsense. It's just a matter of setting the right priorities, and adapting your lifestyle accordingly.

The question is: how important is it to you to look and be fit? Some people just prefer the comfort of a piece of cake and/or a glass of wine in the evening over looking good – whatever makes you happy. Why on earth would you want to work out if it only makes you grumpy?

As far as I'm concerned, looking good is far more important than drinking wine every day and eating things that only pile on the pounds. If you have the same attitude, with careful planning you can also be fit and healthy. Obviously, getting there will take some effort and it is not always easy – even for the likes of me.

Since the establishment of my online platform mykillerbodymotivation.com I work in the office Mondays and Thursdays from 9 a.m. to 6 p.m., on Tuesdays I get off earlier so that I can pick up my son Shai from school, and Wednesday is my day off – my 'mama day'

for going to the cinema or eating out at a nice sushi restaurant. That day is sacred.

I often spend Fridays in my music production studio. It's really handy to have a studio at home as it means I'm never far from Shai, but sometimes I have to go to The Hague and work at my management's studio. On the days I can't pick Shai up, he goes to an after-school club or plays at a friend's house.

When I get home from work in the evening, the last thing I want to do is work out in a crowded gym; I would much rather spend time with my kids and cook them a nice meal, which means I have to get my exercise in before going to work, in the morning. Shai wakes me up at 6.30 a.m., then I help him get dressed, prepare his breakfast and head off to the gym – fortunately it is a stone's throw from where I live so I'm back by 8 a.m., in time to take Shai to school. I must admit I hated that routine at first, but it got better after the first week. Really, you do get used to it. The advantage is also that you get your training out of the way, over and done with, while that extra early start to the day does give you more spare time in the end.

On Saturdays Shai plays football and, while his father attends the away games, I go to all the home games. That can be quite demanding if I've been DJ-ing the night before, but it just makes me so happy.

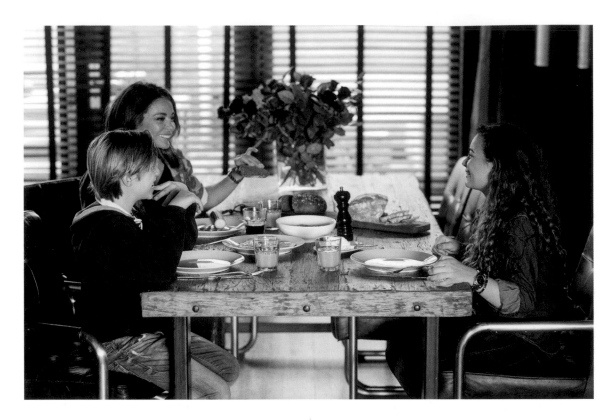

I love both the DJ-ing and seeing my son cavort around the pitch, and that makes it all more than worthwhile even if I do feel extremely tired.

As well as a young son, I have a very independent sixteen-year-old daughter, who really is a great help around the house. And at long last I recently drafted in the services of a cleaning lady who comes once a week. Not that I minded the cobwebs that much, but Shai was getting a bit worried about the spiders!

You can achieve anything in life, as long as it is what you want: a wise lesson my mum always taught me. If you have dreams, write them down. Dreams can become your goals in life, and you can reach those goals. All it takes is a plan, the right kind of support and a positive mindset! Like my mum, I am convinced that everything is possible as long as it is your heart's desire!

How do I keep myself motivated?

You will have bought this book because you felt it was time to get serious about pursuing a healthy, active lifestyle: that was your all-important first step. Now, if you've already done your grocery shop and prepared your meals for the next few days, you are well on your way!

Just to prepare you though, you will probably find this new regime a bit of a breeze in the first few weeks but the novelty does wear off and your motivation will probably start to wane at some point. Having struggled with this myself, I am all too aware how tempting it can be to fall back into those bad old habits.

So here are just a few tips to help you stay on track:

BE REALISTIC

Everyone is different, so don't go comparing yourself to others – especially those beautiful people on Instagram. You may be envious, but those images are only snapshots; we'll never know how much blood, sweat and tears it cost them to get those results. One thing is certain: hardly anyone looks like that naturally (including myself!). Stay focused on your own goals and eventually you will reap the rewards.

KEEP TRACK OF YOUR PROGRESS

The biggest motivating factor will be your own progress, so it's important to keep track of that. Weigh and measure yourself regularly, and take pictures of yourself as well. Write down how you got there – the weights you used, how often you repeated some of the exercises – because once you begin to see how you are reaching your goal, you'll realise why you are doing it and what works for you, and that will strengthen your resolve.

REWARD YOURSELF

My favourite reward for a really tough workout is a cheat meal. Treating yourself after a lot of hard work and achievement is really important as it will give you the incentive to stay with it and persevere. It may not necessarily be food:

perhaps a new sports outfit add that little bit of excitement when you first show it off at the gym? Or how about a nice sports massage after working out? Looking forward to something can really make all the difference.

KEEP TRACK OF WHAT YOU EAT

Feeling you are you not getting anywhere in spite of all your efforts can be a real motivation killer. Keep track of what you eat each day and make sure you are not exceeding your energy requirements; there are some very handy apps for your smartphone to help you.

HAVE SOME FUN

If you're not enjoying your training, you won't be able to keep it up. That is a fact. So choose a form of exercise you enjoy, or at least make whatever you do as much fun as possible: listen to your favourite music, wearing a funky outfit, or persuading a good friend to join you can make all the difference. A gym that has some nice little extras like a sauna, jacuzzi, good showers and a healthy drinks bar can also go a long way.

III
TRAINING

As you've probably guessed by now, it takes more than a little effort to get a **killer body**: aside from a healthy diet, you also need to **train** really hard. And as those who have tried it may already know, sometimes all your best efforts just don't seem to pay off. So in this chapter I will tell you about the **most effective workouts** that will **shape and tone** your body, giving you all the lift you need to **keep going**!

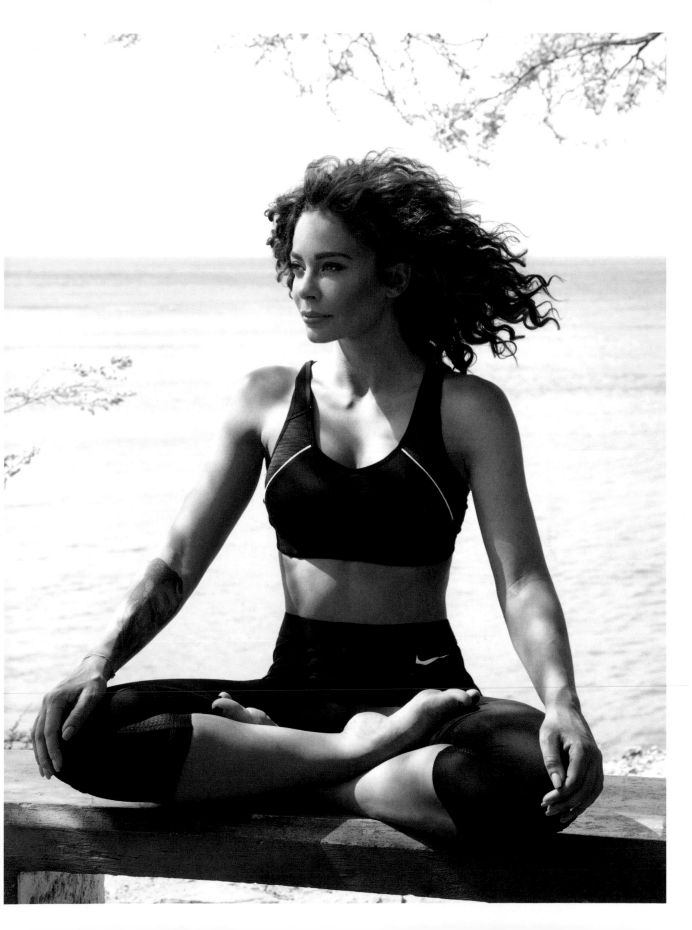

Working the buttocks

Large, round buttocks are now super hot, thanks to celebrities like Kim Kardashian, Beyoncé, Shakira, Jennifer Lopez and other 'curvy women'; so much so that when fashion bible *Vogue* (better known for its skinny, angular models) published an article announcing the arrival of the 'Era of Big Booty' in 2014, it officially became the 'Year of the Butt.' Judging by the compliments I have received for my 'great ass' (thank you very much), I can only say this mirrors my experience. I count myself lucky for having this great asset, a wonderful genetic gift from my mum. But while genes do have a lot to do with it, there are things you can do to improve your rear if you haven't been quite so lucky. And don't forget, even us 'naturals' still have to work hard to keep it all in shape, you know!

'How can I get nice round buttocks and keep my legs from getting bigger as well?' That is a question I'm often asked and the answer is that you need to do exercises that activate the glutes but don't work the legs so hard, like hip thrusts, cable pull-throughs and American deadlifts (ask about these at the gym). It is important to keep increasing the weights rather than doing lots of repetitions with these exercises, because that will really help build your glutes and make them bigger.

The exercises people often do to build nice firm buttocks are squats, lunges and Romanian deadlifts, much of which involves stretching and rotating the hip, and moving the leg out sideways or forward. But while such exercises do activate the glutes, they also work the quadriceps (front of thigh muscle) and hamstrings (back of thigh muscle), and that means your legs will also become more sturdy. Probably not the result you are aiming for if you are a woman.

'YOU CAN'T BUILD NICE ROUND BUTTOCKS WITHOUT INCREASING TRAINING INTENSITY'

If your sole aim is to build firm, round buttocks, you need to make sure you keep exercising those glutes and make your workout increasingly demanding. You can't get nice round buttocks without increasing training intensity, so keep adding more weight and don't stop until your muscles almost give out and you are barely able to finish the exercise. As I said before: it is hard work!

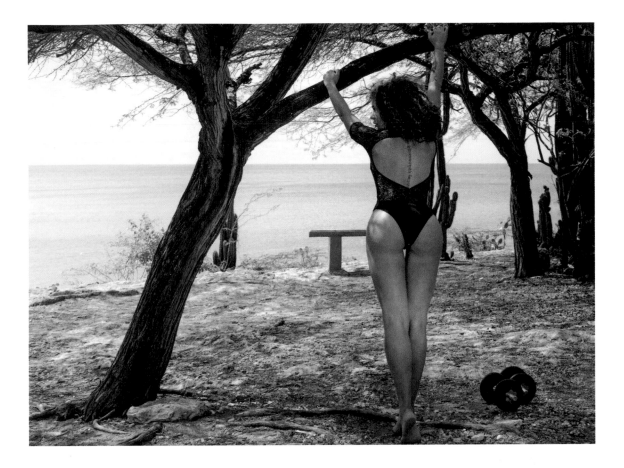

So if you want to go easy on your legs, ask a personal trainer to show you how to do the following exercises, which are specifically for working on the buttocks:

BARBELL GLUTE BRIDGES
You can intensify this exercise by putting your feet on a bench (though this will activate the hamstrings a little more as well) or by also using a barbell, dumbbell or resistance band. Tense your glutes at the most intense part of the movement.

AMERICAN DEADLIFTS
This exercise is better for your glutes than the Romanian deadlift. You can make this as tough as you can bear.

PULL-THROUGHS & KETTLEBELL SWINGS
Make sure you really feel those glutes working during this exercise, and keep tensing them.

SINGLE LEG FOOT ELEVATED HIP THRUST
This one is definitely not for the faint-hearted, but it's very effective. You are bound to see results.

HIP ABDUCTION MOVEMENTS
For example, resistance band seated or standing abduction.

How do I build a nice round bottom?

My shapely rear is a wonderful genetic gift, though it has also taken a fair bit of training. But don't worry if your genes haven't endowed you with the same, there is still hope! Your buttocks consist predominantly of muscle and fat and as we know, muscles can grow and fat can be shed or redistributed. However, it will take rigorous training and a strict, balanced diet.

1 Train your leg muscles and glutes 3 times a week in 6 sets of 6–10 repetitions, using maximum weight. The more weight, the better.

2 Eat plenty of protein; for those who work out regularly, this means 1.8 grams per kilos body weight.

3 Calculate your calorie needs (taking your body type into account):

ECTOMORPH	weight × 44
MESOMORPH	weight × 33
ENDOMORPH	weight × 26

You then increase that amount by 20%, but you've really got to work those glutes or else those additional calories will just turn to extra fat in the places you least want it. But if you do it right, the extra calories will actually help plump up those buttocks!

4 Eating just the right amount for building muscle is tricky, as it is easy to under- or overestimate the amount you need. Use one of those handy apps to keep track of what you eat and check whether you are getting the right amount of calories.

The truth about squats

1 Contrary to popular belief, doing squats exercises your thigh muscles more than your glutes and is therefore not as effective for building shapely, round buttocks.

2 However, squats do form part of a sensible exercise regime because your thigh muscles (quadriceps) form the largest muscle group in your body. Training these muscles stimulates the production of growth hormones, which in turn helps build other muscles.

3 Many women dream of having strong, shapely legs and one of the best exercises to make this happen is the wall sit (sitting on the floor with your back against the wall). The good news is that you can do this practically anywhere, any time, and even watch TV while you're at it! Start with 5 × 30 seconds and gradually build it up, a little more each day, and within a few weeks you will enjoy wearing a snazzy short skirt or dress – if only to show off those killer legs.

Abdominal muscles

Another question people often ask me is: how can I make my abs stand out a bit more? Speaking only from my own experience, my conclusion is that the most important factor in building visible abs is your body fat percentage, which in turn depends on your body type (see page 22). If you fall into the ectomorph category you will find it a lot easier than an endomorph who is relatively more prone to storing fat. I am deliberately avoiding the terms 'six pack' or 'washboard' by the way – for reasons I will explain later.

So it seems then that the first step to well-defined abs would be to get your body fat percentage down. But does it always work? Are visible abs something anyone can achieve? I find that when I gain fat, it goes straight to my thighs, buttocks and triceps (back of the upper arm); my tummy may not always look very tight, but it still looks flat. When, on the other hand, I lose fat my upper body starts to looks a lot tighter, while my legs stay much the same. Even after *Expedition Robinson*, when I lost those 11 kilos, my abs were still absent (see photo on page 7)! Notice also how my face, arms and legs all looked very thin, but my legs were still much the same.

After 5 months of training following the show, while I was no longer thin, I noticed – much to my surprise – that I could actually see my abs, even though I had not done any specific abdominal exercises. I have since realised that when you work your legs very hard, as I tend to do at the gym, you also activate your stomach and core muscles. Just think about it: you can't do squats with 80-kilo weights without standing very strong and stable, and that requires a strong core and strong abdominal muscles. In other words, the harder I trained my legs, the more my abs started to show.

However, this does not take away from the fact that body fat is the key factor in making your abs stand out: you won't see them if they're buried under a layer of fat. But it takes more than simply losing fat for them to be visible, as my story has hopefully demonstrated. Mine only started to show when I began power training, which made me tense my stomach muscles a lot, helping my abs to grow.

'AS YOUR BODY FAT DECREASES, YOUR ABS BECOME MORE VISIBLE'

Again, I am speaking from my own personal experience, of course everyone is different. Whether or not you (can) have fab abs may also depend on your physical traits and genes. Don't forget: exceptions are the rule and there is no point comparing yourself to other people.

Fortunately, there are some general guidelines that may be helpful for developing stronger and more visible abdominal muscles. The first, most important one has already been mentioned: lowering your body fat percentage – in simple terms, losing weight or, if you want to preserve muscle, cutting (see page 86). How much weight you should lose and the right way to do it will depend on your present condition and body type.

Abdominal exercises will only produce visible results if you have lost enough body fat for the muscles to start showing. Nevertheless, doing such exercises is always good to prevent injury and strengthen your core if nothing else. But if the main reason for doing them is to make the muscles more visible, don't be tempted to do hundreds of repetitions, just do slightly more than you would normally do when exercising other muscle groups. Make

'THE HARDER I TRAINED MY LEGS, THE MORE MY ABS STARTED TO SHOW'

sure you add some resistance during the exercises, for example by using weights to the point where you can manage a maximum of 15 to 20 repetitions in succession.

Take care with your breathing whenever you exercise: draw the breath right down into your belly and most importantly, keep breathing. I know it sounds logical, but many people subconsciously hold their breath during (abdominal) exercises so do think about your breathing.

You need a strong core for your abs to show and while power-training will promote that, you can also add some specific exercises that will strengthen the natural function of your core, i.e. stability and anti-rotation (preventing your spine from twisting too far).

A few options are below given (ask a professional trainer to show you how to do these):

- Plank variations, particularly RKC planks
- Farmer Walks/Loaded Carries
- Reverse Crunch (lifting your bottom and lower back off the floor then slowly rolling back down)
- Ab Wheel Roll-outs
- Unilateral leg exercises, like Bulgarian Split Squats
- Stir the Pot
- Split Stance Cable Chops

'ACHIEVING A SIXPACK OR WASHBOARD IS SIMPLY IMPOSSIBLE FOR SOME PEOPLE'

So now the reason I don't like using terms like 'sixpack' or 'washboard': because such an achievement is simply impossible for some people. We all have four stomach muscles and the one down the middle, the rectus abdominis, has either 3 or 4 tendinous intersections, which gives you the potential for either a six- or even eightpack. As the number of tendinous intersections is genetically determined, there is no point trying to get more 'blocks' or change the shape of your rectus abdominis because it just isn't possible.

That's why it's a good idea to get some professional advice on what is achievable for you personally, because you could be wasting your time and efforts if you're doing specific exercises just to make the upper or lower stomach muscles more visible. Besides, research has also shown that the results of such exercises are limited anyway.

How can I get rid of my bingo-wings?

There can't be many women who don't hate bingo-wings, that flabby flesh wobbling underneath your upper arms that is so noticeable when you're waving your child goodbye at the school gates or are wearing a sleeveless dress. But something can be done about those horrors! The muscles at the back of your upper arm, otherwise known as your triceps, can be trained and toned like any other muscle group.

1

Make sure you don't exceed your daily calorie needs. Calculate this on the basis of the following formula, taking your body type into account:

ECTOMORPH	weight × 44
MESOMORPH	weight × 33
ENDOMORPH	weight × 26

2

Train your triceps 3 times a week. You can easily do this at home; the only thing you need is a chair for the dip exercise (see below), and/or a bottle of water.

3

For the dip exercise, start on the floor with your knees bent, arms stretched down, hands flat on the floor pointing towards feet, and then bend and stretch your elbows. Don't count the repetitions, just carry on for as long as you can. Do this 5 times, taking 30-second rests in between.

As soon as you find this is getting too easy, try doing it with straight legs. And if that becomes too easy, put your feet on a chair or bench.

4

Another suitable exercise that you can do at home, even without any weights, is the triceps kickback. Take a bottle of water, bend forward slightly and start moving your bent arm along your body, straightening it as you stretch it backwards. Repeat this as often as you can, doing around 5 rounds for each arm with 30-second rests in between.

5

And finally: push ups. Women often find these the hardest of exercises but you can make it a little easier by resting your knees on the floor. However, do try to push yourself so that eventually you can do it without your knees for support – managing only 2 repetitions without is better than doing none at all! As you are training your triceps, it is crucial that you place your hands only a shoulder-width apart, so that your elbows are almost touching your sides.

Do this exercise as many times as you can. Try 5 rounds as before but with 60-second rests in between. If you do this exercise at least twice (though preferably 3) times per week at home, you'll really notice the difference.

Cardio, good or bad during #MKBM?

I'm not a great fan of cardio, so you're not likely to see me on a cross trainer for longer than the 3 minutes it takes me to warm up. Once upon a time – and only because I had committed to a photoshoot – I did more of it and would spend 20 minutes stepping and then 15 minutes walking on the cross trainer (incline at 15 and speed at 6) after my normal leg exercises. But I don't really run much so I'm not very good at it. What I tend to do after training my upper body is a Tabata workout, which means lots of intervals within a short time: running for 10 seconds on the treadmill, then stopping for 10 seconds, and repeating this 6 times. NOTE: During my Tabata workout the treadmill is turned off so that I have to get it going using my own strength.

Although I'm not that keen on cardio, plenty of people are and mostly because they think it's a great way to burn fat. But while there is truth in that, cardio is in fact not quite as effective as you might think. When you're trying to lose weight, what matters most is your energy balance and, regardless of how much cardio you do, if your energy intake is greater than what you expend you won't lose any weight.

Cardio does burn calories of course but whether you actually lose any fat will depend on how and what you eat, so unfortunately it's no quick fix. What it can do is help improve your metabolism but this will be a very gradual process, so it will still take some perseverance to see any benefit!

One of the less pleasant side-effects of cardio is that it can actually harm your body and strength. If you do cardio alongside power-training you'll find it reduces the benefits of both, which is also known as the 'concurrent training' or 'interference' effect and something you obviously want to avoid. Basically, you're developing your body in 2 different directions because cardio and power-training place very different demands on it. There's a lot of complicated science behind this phenomenon but in simple terms you can compare it to trying to be a sprinter and marathon runner at the same time, when we all know that you can only try to be good at one or the other, not both.

Admittedly, this concurrent training effect is not particularly relevant for people who aren't very active or don't work out a lot. If you're just a beginner, mixing and matching different exercises will not have much adverse impact – at least initially – because your muscles and strength have not yet been finely attuned, so there's no harm in giving it all a try. But developing a killer body is a very specific goal and achieving it will require a much more targeted approach to training.

If you're more advanced, you can try and keep the cardio at a very low or light level to avoid your body adapting to it, but unfortunately you will still not be able to completely eliminate the effects of concurrent training. It is simply impossible to serve 2 masters at once.

'UNFORTUNATELY, CARDIO IS NO QUICK FIX TO BURN FAT'

Bulking

Bulking simply means eating 10–20% more than your body needs to help build muscle. However, do not be tempted to let yourself go and eat whatever junk food and sweets come your way.

Bulking involves a 'controlled increase in food intake' combined with an appropriate training schedule and plenty of rest for the purpose of bringing your body into what is officially called an 'anabolic' state, which 'alerts' your muscles to the fact they have sufficient nutrients for growth.

Preparation

Before you start bulking, you need to make sure you are prepared and well aware of what you're getting into. How much do you really know about power-training? If the answer is 'not a lot', then perhaps ask a personal trainer. Ideally you should also know about proteins, carbohydrates and fats (the macronutrients) because your body fat should remain under 10% of your body weight while you are bulking. Muscle mass won't develop if you gain too much fat and there'd be no point in doing it. So it is crucial to watch what you eat.

The benchmark

The benchmark for determining whether bulking will be beneficial to you is the amount of body fat you have: the higher your body fat percentage at the start of your bulking phase, the more fat your body will store. It is better to start with a low percentage, as your body will then be better prepared for those extra calories. You can measure your body fat percentage with special calipers or get one of the professionals at the gym or your GP to do it for you; if it's higher than 10% and you can't see your upper stomach muscles, you should probably rethink your goals.

Duration

It's difficult to say how long a bulking phase should last. It tends to vary from person to person, depending on how quickly your body fat percentage rises. Generally speaking, it should be around 3 months but you can carry on for longer as long as your body fat percentage stays at an acceptable level, which is why it is so important to keep measuring it regularly (do buy those calipers)! And if your weight goes up while you are bulking, remember to make sure you get the extra energy you need as well.

Step-by-step plan

1 Calculate your energy needs (see the explanation below).
2 Use that as a basis for determining how many additional calories you're going to eat.
3 Determine the right nutrient ratios (see below).
4 Convert calories into grams for each macronutrient (protein, carbohydrate and fat; see explanation below).
5 Divide your total daily calorie intake into 6 or 8 smaller meals and make sure you drink plenty of water.

1 CALCULATE YOUR ENERGY NEEDS

The formula for calculating your daily energy needs is quick and simple: if you know your body type (see page 22) all you need to do is multiply your body weight by the relevant number:

ECTOMORPH	weight × 44
MESOMORPH	weight × 33
ENDOMORPH	weight × 26

Now you need to add your additional energy requirements to take account of your normal daily activity level and the calories you burn in the process. Add the relevant percentage to the basic energy requirement you have just calculated:

+10%	Sedentary job (office, computer work) combined with no training
+20%	Sedentary job combined with light training
+40%	Sedentary job combined with heavy training
+45%	Medium manual labour (a lot of walking; light jobs)
+65%	Medium manual labour combined with heavy training
+70%	Heavy manual labour combined with heavy training

2 CALCULATE YOUR EXTRA DAILY CALORIE NEEDS

So now you have your normal energy needs, to which you can add an additional 200–500 calories for bulking. Don't change your eating pattern overnight, though: slowly build up to the required level and also try and get as many of those extra calories from eating proteins.

Just a little note of caution: even if your bulking diet is exactly right, it's unavoidable that some of the extra calories will still be converted into fat rather than muscle. But if you train hard and your body fat percentage was low to begin with, that effect will be kept to a minimum. However, if you find that your body fat percentage starts to increase too much, just lower your calorie intake for a bit. So once again, you need to keep monitoring your body fat percentage on a regular basis.

3 DETERMINE THE RIGHT NUTRIENT RATIOS

Your extra calories should come from the right balance of proteins, fats and carbohydrates (the macronutrients). You should get this balance right for each meal you eat each day.

The ideal macronutrient ratios for muscle growth are 30% protein, 50% carbohydrates and 20% fats, though it can vary a little from person to person.

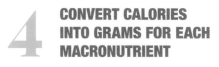

4 CONVERT CALORIES INTO GRAMS FOR EACH MACRONUTRIENT

5 SPREAD YOUR CALORIE INTAKE OVER SEVERAL MEALS

Once you have determined how many grams you need of each of the macronutrients, divide this into 6 or 8 meals per day. That way the food you eat will have a positive effect on your blood sugar and insulin levels, and will help to keep your energy levels up. This is really important because it will ensure that your muscles can repair and grow after training, while you store as little fat as possible.

Just a few more points to mention about bulking:

Regular checks

Checking your diet regularly with a dietitian or personal trainer is advisable because the bulking plan you started out with may not be suitable after a while. For while it can be harmful to keep going for too long, quitting too soon may not give you the results you were aiming for.

Another tip: while you're bulking it's beneficial to combine power- and cardio-training to stay fit and in shape, and to keep your body fat at a constant level.

During your bulking phase you'll want to know if it's actually working so it's a good idea to test your strength from time to time. If you feel you're getting stronger, you're obviously developing more muscle and one look in the mirror should be enough to tell you that they are getting bigger as well.

Eating after training

Obviously, everything you eat throughout the day is important – not only during your bulking phase but afterwards as well – but what matters particularly is that you eat a large meal after exercising. Your body will be craving the right nutrients after a heavy training session so a combination of proteins and fast carbohydrates, such as a big portion of chicken and rice, for example, will be just the ticket. Alternatively, you could also have a protein and dextrose shake straight after training for a quick dose of fast sugars and then have your main meal a little later, once you get home.

Training for maintenance

Once you've finished your bulking phase you may decide to train for maintenance, which means that your calorie intake should match the energy you use up. Figuring out what eating pattern gives you the right balance is basically a case of trial and error. Once you've found this balance your muscles will no longer grow, but neither will you lose muscle as long as you keep training.

1 GRAM PROTEIN = 4 calories
1 GRAM CARBOHYDRATE = 4 calories
1 GRAM FAT = 8 calories

'Cutting'

Cutting simply means eating less to lose fat while preserving muscle through power-training so that you become leaner. When you start cutting, you need to make sure your body fat is at least 8% (you can measure this with special calipers or get it done by a qualified professional at the gym or dietician's practice as explained before) so that you can build muscle even better without losing more fat. To get the best results from cutting, follow these guidelines:

- Calculate your energy needs (see explanation below)
- Stick to a calorie deficit of 200–500 calories
- Determine the right nutrient ratios (percentage of proteins, carbohydrates and fats)
- Convert calories into grams for each macronutrient
- Divide your total calorie requirement by the number of meals you have each day
- Do cardiovascular training (see explanation below)

The formula for calculating your daily energy needs is quick and simple: if you know your body type (see page 22) then all you need to do is multiply your body weight by the relevant number:

ECTOMORPH	weight × 44
MESOMORPH	weight × 33
ENDOMORPH	weight × 26

This will give you the amount of calories you need on a normal day. If you are cutting, take 200–500 calories off this daily requirement. Doing this gradually will help you retain most of your muscle – some loss is unavoidable but the right diet, structural training and plenty of rest should keep that to a minimum.

Take care not to overdo it: if you reduce your carbohydrate intake by 25–50 grams, for example, then you should add back 15–18 grams of protein while keeping your fat intake at the same level to make sure your weight loss is gradual.

The right nutrient ratio

Once you know how many calories you can eat per day during your cutting phase you can simply distribute these calories evenly across your meals. Make sure you stick to precisely the right balance of different macronutrients – when cutting it is generally something like 30% protein, 50% carbohydrates and 20% fat, though it does vary from person to person.

Distribution

While you are cutting, eat at least 6 meals per day and make sure each meal has the right proportion of macronutrients. Spreading the calories over 6 meals will be beneficial for your blood sugar and insulin levels, which will keep your energy levels up, thereby speeding up muscle repair after training and ensuring you store as little fat as possible.

Do cardio training

If cutting is not an option for you or you want to do it less intensively, adding cardio to your training schedule will have the advantage of improving your metabolism. This will help burn more calories even when you're at rest.

I'd advise either a short HIIT (High Intensity Interval Training) workout or a 45-minute cardio session at 70% of your maximum heartrate (ask a professional at the gym to work out your maximum). This is the only way cardio will actually help to burn fat.

Please be aware that cutting calories while doing cardio as well as power-training will put your body through a lot of stress, so make sure you keep plenty of energy to take the strain.

Tips for successful cutting

1 A structured fitness schedule.

2 Eat the right macronutrients (protein, carbohydrates and fat) in the right proportions at the right time.

3 Opt for complex carbohydrates, proteins and healthy fats.

4 Regularly check with a health or fitness professional to see if your training schedule and eating pattern are still appropriate and adapt either or both if necessary.

How much protein do you need while training?

I've already highlighted the importance of macronutrients, and we've looked closely at the reasons why it's important to have the right amounts in the right proportions when you're working out and losing weight. If you're really getting into the Killer Body Plan and you're enjoying the training and active lifestyle, it will probably be useful for you to know a little more about one in particular, namely protein.

Why are proteins so important?

Proteins contain many nutrients and also help to make you feel full, which is an added bonus when you're trying to lose weight by following a strict diet. You also need protein for muscle growth and recovery; for oxygen transportation in the blood; and it's beneficial for your skin and hair as well. Your daily protein requirement will normally depend on your personal situation, body type and weight so if you would like some personal advice on how much protein you need then consult a nutritionist.

The point I really want to highlight here is that some people need more protein than others – children, pregnant women and athletes in particular – but there are a lot of misconceptions about exactly how much, particularly among athletes.

Protein for athletes

Many athletes go by the rule of thumb that to gain muscle you need around 1 gram of protein for every 0.5 kilo of body weight (or, to be more precise: 2.2 grams per kilo). However, research has shown that the positive effect of taking more than 1.8 grams per kilo of body weight is in fact negligible as it won't give you more muscle growth, no matter how hard you train. So this rule is basically a myth; the idea that the more active you are the more protein you need – as many athletes seem to believe – is in fact nonsense!

'THE MORE YOU TRAIN, THE MORE EFFICIENTLY YOUR BODY BREAKS DOWN THE PROTEINS'

Nevertheless, the sports community still tends to adhere to the 2.2 grams protein rule, with many athletes still thinking they need more protein to enable them to train hard. But it really doesn't hold true: one research study even concluded that experienced bodybuilders actually need less protein than beginners, and these findings have been supported by several other studies as well. The reason is that the more you train the smarter your body gets at breaking down the proteins so that in fact you need less and less to achieve good muscle growth. And even aside from that, there is such a thing as a 'genetic limit': everyone has a maximum amount of muscle they can gain and as you approach that limit muscle growth will slow down, so reducing your need for protein. Makes sense, doesn't it?

'CHILDREN, PREGNANT WOMEN AND ATHLETES NEED EXTRA PROTEIN'

Protein intake while cutting

Nevertheless, quite a number of athletes remain convinced that when you are cutting you need that 2.2 grams of daily protein (for more info on cutting see page 86). But again, research findings do not support this: the overwhelming evidence points to 1.8 grams per kilo of body weight being sufficient. One study had people running on heavy training schedules and a protein deficit of 1000 calories; even then, 1.8 grams of protein was found to be sufficient to prevent muscle loss.

In short: there is no empirical evidence to suggest that if you are an athlete you need more than 1.8 grams of protein per kilo of body weight every day. However, that is not to say that it would be wrong to consume more than is needed for building muscle because your body will simply store the surplus for extra energy. But the consequence of that is that you'll obviously need to work harder to make sure you use up that extra energy, just to avoid gaining weight.

Protein shakes

Protein, as we all know, is a vital nutrient – especially when you're doing a lot of training and/or following a diet – so it's hardly surprising that protein powder is not difficult to come by. In fact, you can find it almost anywhere, certainly in health food shops and online. But there are different kinds of protein so you may be asking yourself: which one is best and, moreover, for what purpose? There are plenty of recipes for cakes or banana bread online but they hardly ever tell you specifically what proteins to use. So just in case you're wondering, let me shed some more light on this.

Before I delve into the subject a little more, let me tell you how and when I take protein powder myself and the reasons why. I take it, first of all, when I'm going through one of my heavy training phases and am sticking to a very strict diet. That's when I start the day with my protein-powder pancakes (recipe on page 168).

The only other time I resort to taking it is during a cutting phase when I'm eating fewer calories than I need to try and lose fat. Although I'm deliberately eating less, I really hate going to sleep with that hungry feeling so a casein protein shake before bed readily solves that problem (I'll discuss the different types of protein later on).

It obviously doesn't help me lose weight but at least it's a quick and safe way of feeling full when I'm off to bed. And here's another handy little tip: sometimes I turn my protein shake into a scrumptious dessert just by adding a teaspoon of raw cocoa and a tablespoon of peanut butter. It tastes like a Snickers bar, in liquid form! But do watch out, the tablespoon of peanut butter actually contains 100 calories so check it doesn't tip you over your daily calorie limit.

'I TURN MY PROTEIN SHAKE INTO A SCRUMPTIOUS DESSERT JUST BY ADDING A TEASPOON OF RAW COCOA AND A TABLESPOON OF PEANUT BUTTER'

Iso, whey or casein?

So now the theory bit about protein shakes. There are 3 varieties – iso, whey and casein – and I often get asked which one is best. It depends on the reason for having it: casein is 'slow' protein, which helps stave off the hunger for longer. But if you've just finished training, you'd be better off choosing whey because that will refuel your muscles more quickly.

There are a number of different ways of ensuring you get the right amount of protein. Eating some of those protein pancakes I mentioned earlier, for example – though it's worth noting that whey proteins are actually destroyed in the process of heating so bear that in mind when you're using it in hot food. So let me tell you a little more about whey and casein proteins, and the difference between them . . .

Casein is the main protein present in milk and (in coagulated form) in cheese; whey is the watery part of milk that remains after the formation of curds. The amino acids in whey differ from those in casein – and remember that amino acids are the building blocks of proteins. You can read more about this in the chapter on BCAA and other nutritional supplements (see page 60).

It's difficult to say which type of protein is better for you. If your muscles are crying out for a quick refuel after exercise, it's best to go for whey because it's a much faster acting protein. But casein will raise the amino acids much more slowly and for a longer period as well, which is better when you're on a diet, for example.

This is why each of the 3 phases of the beginner's diet in this book include a late-night casein-based snack (a casein shake during the first 2 phases), to help you get to sleep feeling nice and full. As you sleep, the casein will also be refuelling your muscles so they can recover and grow. Your body produces growth hormones while you rest as well, which is also very important for muscle development. Casein supports this process and will help you get the most out of all that hard work at the gym.

So if you're going to experiment with taking extra protein, do make sure you know why you're taking it and use the right type in the most suitable form, i.e. decide whether it should be something cold/hot/liquid or solid.

Finally, the third protein is iso – short for isolate – which is in fact the purest type of protein. Although you might regard it as a protein concentrate, it is not quite the same as a concentrate has other added substances which reduce its protein content; an isolate has at least 90% protein and therefore fewer fats and carbohydrates. There are whey- as well as casein-isolates on the market.

Alcohol and training

My Killer Body diet doesn't feature any alcohol, but if you're anything like me you probably enjoy a good party and having a drink or two. So let me assure you that there is no need to become a teetotaller to get a killer body. It is actually even possible to drink alcohol and still burn fat, with minimal impact on your training. Yes, really! It all has to do with the way your body processes the alcohol.

Alcohol enters the blood stream via your stomach and intestines, and then the liver breaks it down into acetic acid (acetate), which puts the brakes on fat loss as soon as it enters the bloodstream. As a result, your body then stores most of the fatty acids in your blood and so you put on weight – and potentially end up with that tell-tale beer belly.

But it's not all bad news. The fact is that less than 5% of the alcohol you drink is turned into fat; your body isn't very efficient in converting the acetate into fat and your liver is far too busy breaking it down to produce its own. Furthermore – and this may be a pleasant surprise for some of you – alcohol itself contains no fat at all, and very few carbohydrates. So if your body has very little fat before you start drinking the effect of alcohol can be minimised.

So it's not the alcohol itself that makes you fat (though it obviously does contains calories, around 7 calories per gram) but the way in which your body reacts to it, as it makes your body store fat. But this is the kind of knowledge we can turn to our advantage; there are ways to get around the effects of alcohol:

'IT'S NOT THE ALCOHOL ITSELF THAT MAKES YOU FAT'

1 Eat as little fat as possible on the days you drink so that your body has little or no fat to store.

2 Leave as much time as possible between your training session and drinking. Recent research has shown a direct link between alcohol consumption and reduced muscle development so it's best not to go training right before a party. It is better to go first thing in the morning or perhaps not at all.

3 Take it steady when you're drinking: don't binge, as this will give you a sudden energy boost prompting your body to react by storing the surplus.

4 Eat less when you're drinking to make sure you keep within your daily calorie limit. That will also help you feel the effects of alcohol – and get drunk, if that is the effect you are after – more quickly.

5 Do eat a lot of carbs and especially proteins right before you start drinking as these will counter the effects of alcohol in various ways. A full stomach slows the rate of absorption of alcohol into the blood so that some of it will be broken down in your stomach by the enzymes from the food you have eaten, giving your liver more time to break down the alcohol before it enters the bloodstream. A hearty meal, containing a lot of slow proteins and fibre, can as much as halve the damaging effects of alcohol.

6 Drink only wine, champagne or vodka as they contain the least amount of sugar. Beer is the worst as it normally contains more than 200 calories per pint.

7 If you tend to get peckish and are unable to resist a snack after drinking (another effect of alcohol), make sure that you eat fewer calories during the day and have a hearty meal with lots of protein ready and waiting for you when you get home.

IV

DIET PLAN & TRAINING SCHEDULES

Diet for a killer body
Diet plan
Training home workout
Effective training:
variation in focus
Training at the gym

Diet for a killer body

DIET PLAN

Note: If you have more than 24% body fat you should start with Phase 1 of the diet. We won't be counting calories during those first 12 weeks; the diet is designed to ensure you get all the right nutrition and protein you need to retain muscle. Even if your aim is to get leaner, you should start with Phase 1 if your body fat is higher than 24%.

If your body fat is below that level and you work out at least 4–5 times a week to gain muscle mass, you can start with the sports diet. This diet is not necessarily a continuation of the beginner's diet – which is aimed at losing weight – but specifically tailored to the requirements of the active athlete whose purpose is muscle growth.

So let's get started! The following pages will outline the 3 phases of my diet that will set you on course to a killer body. But just to emphasise once more: the beginner's diet is aimed at people who are overweight. Unless you're an active, experienced athlete – in which case the sports diet will be more suitable – it is always best to start on this diet. Then, once you have lost sufficient weight you can go back to Phase 1 and keep following that to maintain your target weight, and even gradually start eating a little more as long as you keep within your daily calorie limit. The second and third phases are really designed for weight loss only.

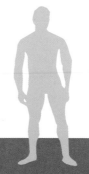

NOTE!

The diet below was created with women in mind: men should add one slice of wholemeal bread, 30 grams of meat or fish and 50 grams of rice, pasta or potatoes to the daily portions.

'IF YOU WANT TO LOSE WEIGHT, YOU HAVE TO EMBRACE THOSE HUNGER PANGS'

A tailor-made diet plan

If, once you have lost sufficient weight you want to start growing muscle or become leaner I would advise a tailor-made diet plan. My website **mykillerbodymotivation. com** gives all the information you need to devise your own plan, as well as the option to request one created especially for you by one of the coaches I work with.

Substitution list

If any of the foods in the diet are not to your taste or cause problems (e.g. you have allergies), feel free to change it for another food from the list of substitutes on page 205. However, do take care you choose an equivalent product , i.e. one that contains the same macronutrients. So if you want to swap a protein-rich food, choose something that is equally rich in protein; the same applies to foods that are high in fats or carbohydrates. Chicken, which is rich in protein is obviously no substitute for bread, which is high in carbohydrates. The list of substitutes is there to guide you in making your choice.

Shopping lists

It can be really challenging, sticking to my diet – any diet, for that matter – so make it as easy as possible for yourself, for instance by making sure your larder is always well stocked up (that is one of my tactics). The shopping lists in this book (from page 204) are there to get you started; there is one for every dieting phase, each lasting 4 weeks. It will certainly help ensure you get all the groceries you need, making it less likely that you'll stray from your diet.

Every phase lasts 4 weeks, enabling your body to get used to your new eating pattern. It's really important that you stay with each phase for the whole duration to get the best results.

Phase one

The first phase is designed to get you used to eating regular meals and cutting out the unhealthy sugars. Be warned: at times you will feel hungry but that's exactly the point. If you want to lose weight, you have to embrace those hunger pangs.

You will start craving more food because you won't be meeting your normal daily calorie needs but by doing this your body will be forced to use up fat reserves as you keep up your daily activity level. If you start to feel faint, just have some fat-free broth.

Eating more fruit than the diet prescribes is not an option, but if your hunger is really getting the better of you have an extra portion of vegetables or any other product that can be eaten without restriction.

If at any time you need a little extra just to keep going, you can always pick something from the list below, which you can have whenever you need a little pick-me-up:

- **Boiled or grilled vegetables (no limit)**
- Cucumber with a pinch of salt
- 2 tomatoes
- Radishes
- Either 1 rice cake or
- 1 light cracker a day
- 2 boiled eggs

Phase two

During this phase you'll be eating a lot of carbs one day and then hardly any on the next, a pattern referred to as 'Carb Cycling'. You should really stick to this pattern as it's a very effective way to get all the carbohydrates you need while storing as little fat as possible. It will give you all the 'joys' – i.e. the energy you need – without suffering the 'downs' (low energy, bad moods) on the days you eat fewer carbs. It will be important, however, to:

- Train on the days you eat more carbs so that your body gets the maximum benefit, and the energy obtained is used for training or recovery.
- Keep protein intake at the same level throughout (both on training and non-training days).
- Don't give up part-way through this second phase of the diet, even if you're disappointed with the results. Your body simply needs a little time to adjust to this new eating pattern; remember that consistency is the key to achievement.

If you feel you haven't lost enough weight after 4 weeks, just follow Phase 2 of the diet for another 4 weeks.

Phase three

During this phase, you'll be eating very little for 6 days and then have a refeed every Sunday, eating 3 meals with extra carbs (more about this on page 51). If you've managed to get down to your target weight after completing this phase, you can carry on eating as you did during Phase 1 to maintain that weight. Do read page 46 first, however, to calculate your basic daily calorie needs.

I maintain my weight by Intermittent Fasting (IF) 2 days a week; you can read more about this on page 55.

You can start Phase 1 of the diet either at the same time as Phase 1 of the training schedule or leave it until later after you've started training.

PHASE 1 WEEK 1–4

	TIME *(personal choice)*	MONDAY	TUESDAY	WEDNESDAY
BREAKFAST		200 ml Greek yogurt, 0% fat 1 teaspoon cinnamon ½ apple	omelette made with 1 whole egg and 2 egg whites 1 toasted slice of wholemeal bread	protein pancake (p. 168)
SNACK 1		½ cucumber with a pinch of salt and cinnamon	1 small wholegrain bread roll with peanut butter (10 g)	100 g cottage cheese with cinnamon
LUNCH		wholemeal wrap (40 g) ¼ avocado 80 g grilled chicken breast lettuce, tomato and cucumber	2 light crackers 10 g houmous 4 slices chicken breast 150 g low-fat Quark with cinnamon	tuna salad (p. 170)
SNACK 2		1 apple with cinnamon	1 apple with cinnamon	1 orange
DINNER		80 g uncooked rice (cook before eating) 100 g chicken breast stir-fry vegetables with soy sauce for added flavour lettuce, cucumber and tomato with a dash of salt, pepper and lemon	80 g sweet potato 100 g white fish 5 large asparagus lettuce, cucumber and tomato	spicy penne and smoked trout (p. 192)
LATE NIGHT SNACK		casein protein shake (see also p. 90) dosage: 2 level scoops (just over 30 g) www.MKBMshop.com Enter code: MKBMproteine for a 10% discount	casein protein shake dosage: 2 level scoops (just over 30 g)	casein protein shake dosage: 2 level scoops (just over 30 g)

DRINK PLENTY OF WATER! (2.5–3.5 LITRES A DAY)

Water plays an important role in lipid metabolism. It is essential for the conversion of fat into energy, reduces appetite, alleviates constipation and helps remove waste from the body, which in turn, helps keep energy levels up.

PHASE 1 WEEK 1–4

THURSDAY	FRIDAY	SATURDAY		SUPPS
				(1 × daily)
overnight oats (p. 166)	200 g low-fat (flavoured) Quark	protein pancake (p. 168)	2 fried eggs 1 tomato ½ cucumber 30 g cottage cheese	1 BCAA multivitamin, fish oil, vitamin D
1 apple with cinnamon	omelette made with 1 whole egg and 2 egg whites ½ apple with cinnamon	½ cucumber with pinch of salt 30 g cottage cheese	1 apple with cinnamon	
80 g steak tartare 2 light crackers 2 boiled eggs	wholemeal wrap (40 g) 50 g smoked salmon iceberg lettuce 10 g cream light cheese capers (optional)	chicken salad (p. 172)	2 light crackers 30 g cottage cheese 4 slices chicken breast 2 slices tomato	
½ avocado with salt and pepper	fat-free broth 1 breadstick	1 apple with cinnamon	200 g low-fat Quark 1 teaspoon honey cocoa powder (optional)	
80 g uncooked rice (cook before eating) 100 g lean ground beef runner beans, onion and garlic	courgette spaghetti and cream cheese (p. 182)	80 g uncooked rice (cook before eating) 100 g white fish 200 g broccoli	veggie salad (p. 174)	
casein protein shake dosage: 2 level scoops (just over 30 g)	casein protein shake dosage: 2 level scoops (just over 30 g)	casein protein shake dosage: 2 level scoops (just over 30 g)	casein protein shake dosage: 2 level scoops (just over 30 g)	

MEN

For men add: 1 slice of bread, 30 g meat or fish and 50 g uncooked rice, pasta or potatoes.

PHASE 2 WEEK 5–8

TIME *(personal choice)*	MONDAY	TUESDAY	WEDNESDAY
BREAKFAST	30 g porridge ½ banana 1 teaspoon cinnamon 20 g whey protein mix with water	200 g low-fat Quark 1 teaspoon honey	1 slice toasted wholemeal bread 30 g smoked beef
SNACK 1	2 rice cakes ¼ avocado 4 slices chicken breast	½ avocado pinch of salt	1 light cracker 30 g cottage cheese 4 slices chicken breast
LUNCH	40 g wholemeal wrap 50 g smoked chicken breast 2 slices tomato lettuce boiled egg	veggie salad (p. 174)	1 slice wholemeal bread 6 slices chicken breast boiled egg
SNACK 2	1 apple with cinnamon	3 pineapple slices	1 apple with cinnamon
DINNER	80 g wholemeal pasta homemade Bolognese sauce (p. 184) courgette, onions, garlic 75 g lean ground beef	oven-baked chicken (p. 186)	80 g uncooked rice (cook before eating) 200 g stir-fried mixed vegetables, 100 g fried shrimps or chicken 1 teaspoon soy sauce salt, pepper, garlic
LATE NIGHT SNACK	casein protein shake dosage: 2 level scoops (just over 30 g) www.MKBMshop.com Enter code: MKBMproteine for a 10% discount	casein protein shake dosage: 2 level scoops (just over 30 g)	casein protein shake dosage: 2 level scoops (just over 30 g)

DRINK PLENTY OF WATER! (2.5–3.5 LITRES A DAY)

Water plays an important role in lipid metabolism. It is essential for the conversion of fat into energy, reduces appetite, alleviates constipation and helps remove waste from the body, which in turn, helps keep energy levels up.

PHASE 2 WEEK 5–8

THURSDAY	FRIDAY	SATURDAY	SUNDAY	SUPPS
				(1 × daily)
omelette made with 1 whole egg and 2 egg whites spinach salt and pepper 1 slice wholemeal bread	protein pancake (p. 168)	2 fried eggs 4 slices chicken breast 2 slices tomato 2 breadsticks	wholemeal wrap (40 g) 50 g chicken breast 1 tomato ½ cucumber	1 BCAA multivitamin, fish oil, vitamin D
1 apple with cinnamon	2 rice cakes 1 tablespoon of houmous 4 slices chicken breast	200 g low-fat flavoured Quark	1 apple with cinnamon	
tuna salad (p. 170) 2 breadsticks 1 kiwi fruit	1 slice wholemeal bread 50 g smoked meat 1 kiwi fruit	80 g mozzarella light 1 tomato 1 teaspoon pesto salt and pepper pumpkin soup (p. 178)	vegetarian lasagne (p. 182)	
3 slices of pineapple	1 apple with cinnamon	1 orange	200 g low-fat Quark 5 walnuts 1 teaspoon honey	
100 g lean ground beef (meatballs) 200 g green beans ½ cucumber 1 tomato	80 g sweet potato 100 g white fish 200 g vegetables season with salt, pepper and lemon	100 g grilled chicken breast 200 g broccoli salad without dressing	homemade burger (p. 188)	
casein protein shake dosage: 2 level scoops (just over 30 g)	casein protein shake dosage: 2 level scoops (just over 30 g)	casein protein shake dosage: 2 level scoops (just over 30 g)	casein protein shake dosage: 2 level scoops (just over 30 g)	

MEN

For men add: 1 slice wholemeal bread, 30 g meat or fish and 50 g uncooked rice, pasta or potatoes.

PHASE 3 WEEK 9–12

	TIME *(personal choice)*	MONDAY	TUESDAY	WEDNESDAY
BREAKFAST		1 slice toasted wholemeal bread 30 g smoked meat 30 g cottage cheese	protein pancake (p. 168) 100 g low-fat Quark 1 teaspoon honey	omelette made with 1 whole egg and 3 egg whites fresh spinach fry in coconut oil
SNACK 1		2 kiwi fruits 1 fat-free broth 2 breadsticks	1 orange	1 small wholegrain bread roll with butter
LUNCH		green soup (p. 180) breadstick ½ cucumber	chicken salad (p. 172)	100 g carpaccio rocket 10 g pine nuts 1 breadstick
SNACK 2		2 rice cakes 1 tablespoon peanut butter ½ cucumber	150 g low-fat yogurt 30 g muesli	1 apple with cinnamon
DINNER		chicken salad (p. 172) 2 breadsticks	80 g uncooked rice (cook before eating) 75 g shrimp/white fish 200 g stir-fry vegetables fry in coconut oil	80 g wholemeal pasta 75 g lean ground beef, homemade Bolognese sauce (p. 184) lettuce, cucumber without dressing
LATE NIGHT SNACK		casein protein shake dosage: 2 level scoops (just over 30 g) 1 teaspoon peanut butter www.MKBMshop.com Enter code: MKBMproteine for a 10% discount	casein protein shake dosage: 2 level scoops (just over 30 g) 1 teaspoon peanut butter	casein protein shake dosage: 2 level scoops (just over 30 g) 1 teaspoon peanut butter

DRINK PLENTY OF WATER! (2.5–3.5 LITRES A DAY)

Water plays an important role in lipid metabolism. It is essential for the conversion of fat into energy, reduces appetite, alleviates constipation and helps remove waste from the body, which in turn, helps keep energy levels up.

PHASE 3 WEEK 9–12

THURSDAY	FRIDAY	SATURDAY	SUNDAY	SUPPS
				(1 × daily)
150 g low-fat Quark 2 dates, 3 walnuts 1 kiwi fruit	2 light crackers 30 g chicken breast 30 g cottage cheese 4 slices tomato	1 small wholegrain bread roll with butter 2 boiled eggs	3 fried eggs 30 g chicken breast 30 g cottage cheese 2 slices wholemeal bread	1 BCAA multivitamin, fish oil, vitamin D
2 light crackers 30 g cottage cheese 4 slices tomato	1 apple with cinnamon	150 g low-fat Quark 1 teaspoon honey	1 banana 200 g low-fat Quark 40 g porridge	
protein pancake (p. 168) 1 kiwi fruit	1 slice toasted wholemeal bread 70 g roast beef	tuna salad (p. 170) 1 breadstick	2 wholemeal wraps (40 g each) 60 g chicken breast (sliced) 30 g cottage cheese iceberg lettuce	
50 g smoked fish or 2 herrings	1 orange	1 kiwi fruit	1 small wholegrain bread roll with butter	
80 g sweet potato 100 g chicken breast 200 g green vegetables fry in coconut oil	80 g uncooked rice (cook before eating) 75 g lean ground beef, season with onion, garlic and some salt 200 g runner beans	oven-baked chicken (p. 186)	burger and bun (p. 188) lettuce 10 french fries	
casein protein shake dosage: 2 level scoops (just over 30 g) 1 teaspoon peanut butter	casein protein shake dosage: 2 level scoops (just over 30 g) 1 teaspoon peanut butter	casein protein shake dosage: 2 level scoops (just over 30 g) 1 teaspoon peanut butter	casein protein shake dosage: 2 level scoops (just over 30 g) 30 g porridge ½ banana	

MEN

Men can add 1 slice wholemeal bread and 30 g meat or fish to this diet.

PHASE 1 SPORTS DIET WEEK 1–4

	TIME *(personal choice)*	MONDAY	TUESDAY	WEDNESDAY
BREAKFAST		30–50 g porridge 3–4 strawberries 1 kiwi fruit 30–50 g whey isolate 1 tablespoon linseed oil	omelette made with 2 whole eggs and 4–7 egg whites handful of spinach	200 ml Greek yogurt 0% fat 8–10 blueberries 40–70 g porridge ½ banana 30–50 g whey protein
SNACK 1		2–4 rice cakes 150 g white fish 150 g cooked or raw vegetables	1 tomato ½ cucumber 140 g tinned tuna (in water)/white fish 1 tablespoon olive oil	100 g chicken breast ½ avocado red/green pepper
LUNCH		BLEND: handful of spinach 150 ml almond milk juice of ½ lemon ½ avocado 30–50 g whey protein	100 g uncooked brown rice (cook before eating) 100 g chicken breast 20 g walnuts raw vegetables of your choice	100 g uncooked brown rice (cook before eating) 100 g chicken breast 150–200 g cooked or raw vegetables
SNACK 2		100 g uncooked brown rice (cook before eating) 150 g chicken breast lettuce, cucumber, tomato, onion	30–50 g whey protein 2 rice cakes with peanut butter (15 g)	100 g white fish 150–200 green vegetables 1 boiled egg
DINNER		100–150 g steak/steak tartare mushrooms	100 g uncooked brown rice (cook before eating) 150 g white fish lettuce, cucumber, tomato, onion	50 g wholemeal pasta 150 g chicken breast 150 g broccoli 1 pineapple slice
LATE NIGHT SNACK		omelette made with 5–8 egg whites 1 green apple 30 g nuts (unsalted) www.MKBMshop.com Enter code: MKBMproteine for a 10% discount	20 g walnuts 40–50 g casein protein	30 g almonds 200 g cottage cheese 1 pineapple slice

DRINK PLENTY OF WATER! (2.5–3.5 LITRES A DAY)

Water plays an important role in lipid metabolism. It is essential for the conversion of fat into energy, reduces appetite, alleviates constipation and helps remove waste from the body, which in turn, helps keep energy levels up.

PHASE 1 SPORTS DIET WEEK 1–4

THURSDAY	FRIDAY	SATURDAY	SUNDAY	SUPPS
				(1 × daily)
50–90 g porridge 3–4 strawberries 1 kiwi fruit 30–50 g whey isolate 1 tablespoon linseed oil	omelette made with 2 whole eggs and 4–7 egg whites handful of spinach	200 ml Greek yogurt 0% fat 8–10 blueberries 70–120 g porridge ½ banana 30–50 g whey protein	50–90 g porridge 3–4 strawberries 1 kiwi fruit 30–50 g whey isolate 1 tablespoon linseed oil	1 BCAA multivitamin, fish oil, vitamin D
2–4 rice cakes 100 g white fish 150 g cooked or raw vegetables	1 tomato ½ cucumber 100 g of tinned tuna (in water)/white fish 1 tablespoon olive oil	100 g chicken breast ½ avocado red/green pepper	2–4 rice cakes 100 g white fish 150 g cooked or raw vegetables	
BLEND: handful of spinach 150 ml almond milk juice of ½ lemon ½ avocado 30–50 g whey protein	100 g uncooked brown rice (cook before eating) 100 g chicken breast 20 g walnuts raw vegetables of your choice	100 g uncooked brown rice (cook before eating) 100 g chicken breast 150–200 g cooked or raw vegetables	BLEND: handful of spinach 150ml almond milk juice of ½ lemon ½ avocado 30–50 g whey protein	
100 g uncooked brown rice (cook before eating) 100 g chicken breast lettuce, cucumber, tomato, onion	30–50 g whey protein 2 rice cakes with peanut butter (15 g)	100 g white fish 150–200 green vegetables 1 boiled egg	100 g uncooked brown rice (cook before eating) 100 g chicken breast lettuce, cucumber, tomato, onion	
100 g steak/steak tartare mushrooms	100 g uncooked brown rice (cook before eating) 100 g white fish lettuce, cucumber, tomato, onion	100 g wholemeal pasta 150 g chicken breast 150 g broccoli 1 pineapple slice	100–150 g steak / steak tartare mushrooms	
omelette made with 5–8 egg whites 1 green apple 30 g nuts (unsalted)	20 g walnuts 40–50 g casein protein	30 g almonds 200 ml cottage cheese 1 pineapple slice	omelette made with 5–8 egg whites 1 green apple 30 g nuts (unsalted)	

MEN

Men who are following this plan can add 100 g meat, 100 g carbohydrates and 2 slices of wholemeal bread to the diet.

PHASE 2 SPORTS DIET WEEK 5–8

	TIME *(personal choice)*	MONDAY	TUESDAY	WEDNESDAY
BREAKFAST		50–75 g cereal 30–50 g whey isolate 20 g raisins 20 g almonds	handful of spinach 1 kiwi fruit juice of ½ lemon ¼ avocado 30–50 g whey protein 150 ml almond milk	50–75 g porridge ½ banana 1 kiwi fruit 30–50 g whey isolate 20 g walnuts
SNACK 1		150 g chicken breast 1 pineapple slice cucumber	100–120 g salmon or mackerel 100 g raw vegetables of your choice 2–4 rice cakes	150 g chicken breast 1 green apple with cinnamon 4 rice cakes
LUNCH		30–50 g whey protein 2 rice cakes with peanut butter (15 g)	100 g uncooked Basmati rice (cook before eating) 150 g chicken breast 150–200 g vegetables of your choice	100 g uncooked Basmati rice (cook before eating) 150 g fish of your choice 150–200 g cooked or raw vegetables
SNACK 2		100 g uncooked Basmati rice (cook before eating) 150 g white fish lettuce, cucumber, tomato, onion	150–200 g low-fat Quark 80 g pineapple in its own juice or with cinnamon	30–50 g cereal 30–40 g whey protein 20 g raisins
DINNER		1 fried egg 150 g chicken breast or steak 150 g green beans	100 g uncooked Basmati rice (cook before eating) 100–150 g chicken breast 150–200 g green vegetables	100 g uncooked Basmati rice (cook before eating) 100–150 g steak/steak tartare 150 g broccoli 1 pineapple slice
LATE NIGHT SNACK		250–500 g low-fat Quark 8–10 blueberries 20 g walnuts www.MKBMshop.com Enter code: MKBMproteine for a 10% discount	1 egg 40–50 g casein protein 8–10 blueberries	30–50 g casein protein 20 g almonds

DRINK PLENTY OF WATER! (2.5–3.5 LITRES A DAY)

Water plays an important role in lipid metabolism. It is essential for the conversion of fat into energy, reduces appetite, alleviates constipation and helps remove waste from the body, which in turn, helps keep energy levels up.

PHASE 2 SPORTS DIET WEEK 5–8

THURSDAY	FRIDAY	SATURDAY	SUNDAY	SUPPS
				(1 × daily)
50–75 g cereal 30–50 g whey isolate 20 g raisins 20 g almonds	handful of spinach 1 kiwi fruit juice of ½ lemon ¼ avocado 30–50 g whey protein 150 ml almond milk	75–125 g porridge ½ banana 1 kiwi fruit 30–50 g whey isolate 20 g walnuts	50–75 g cereal 30–50 g whey isolate 20 g raisins 20 g almonds	1 BCAA multivitamin, fish oil, vitamin D
150 g chicken breast 1 pineapple slice cucumber	100–120 g salmon or mackerel 100 g raw vegetables of your choice 2–4 rice cakes	150 g chicken breast 1 green apple with cinnamon 4 rice cakes	150 g chicken breast 1 pineapple slice cucumber	
30–50 g whey protein 2 rice cakes with peanut butter (15 g)	100 g uncooked Basmati rice (cook before eating) 150 g chicken breast 150–200 g vegetables of your choice	100 g uncooked Basmati rice (cook before eating) 150 g fish of your choice 150–200 g cooked or raw vegetables	30–50 g whey protein 2 rice cakes with peanut butter (15 g)	
100 g uncooked Basmati rice (cook before eating) 150 g white fish lettuce, cucumber, tomato, onion	250–500 g of low-fat Quark 80 g pineapple in its own juice or with cinnamon	30–50 g cereal 30–40 g whey protein 20 g raisins	100 g uncooked Basmati rice (cook before eating) 150 g white fish lettuce, cucumber, tomato, onion	
1 fried egg 150 g chicken breast or steak 150 g green beans	100 g uncooked Basmati rice (cook before eating) 100–150 g chicken breast 150–200 g green vegetables	100 g uncooked Basmati rice (cook before eating) 100–150 g steak/steak tartare 150 g broccoli 1 pineapple slice	1 fried egg 150 g chicken breast or steak 150 g green beans	
250–500 g low-fat Quark 8–10 blueberries 20 g walnuts	1 egg 40–50 g casein protein 8–10 blueberries	30–50 g casein protein 20 g almonds	250–500 g low-fat Quark 8–10 blueberries 20 g walnuts	

www.MKBMshop.com
Enter code:
MKBMproteine for
a 10% discount

MEN

Men who follow this nutrition plan can add 100 g meat to the diet.

PHASE 3 SPORTS DIET WEEK 9–12

	TIME *(personal choice)*	MONDAY	TUESDAY	WEDNESDAY
BREAKFAST		omelette made with 2 whole eggs and 4–6 egg whites 1 slice toasted wholemeal bread 1 tomato	50–70 g porridge 10–12 blueberries ½ banana 30–50 g whey isolate	50–75 g cereal 20 g raisins 20 g walnuts 30–50 g whey protein
SNACK 1		150 g chicken breast 1 green apple with cinnamon	50 g chicken breast 3–4 egg whites 2–4 rice cakes ½ cucumber	2 slices wholemeal bread 100 g chicken breast 1 egg
LUNCH		100 g uncooked Basmati rice (cook before eating) 150 g chicken breast 150–200 g vegetables of your choice	100 g uncooked Basmati rice (cook before eating) 150 g white fish 20 g almonds 100–150 g raw vegetables	100–150 g raw vegetables ¼ avocado 150 g smoked chicken breast/salmon carpaccio
SNACK 2		30–50 g whey protein 2 rice cakes with peanut butter (15 g)	100 g roast beef 2–4 rice cakes 1 apple	100 g wholemeal pasta 100–150 g steak tartare tomato sauce Italian vegetable mix
DINNER		50 g uncooked Basmati rice (cook before eating) 150 g white fish 150–200 g stir-fry vegetables 1 pineapple slice	50 g uncooked brown rice (cook before eating) 150 g chicken breast 200 g stir-fry vegetables 1 tablespoon olive oil	2 rice cakes 80–100 g chicken breast ½ cucumber
LATE NIGHT SNACK		150–250 g low-fat Quark 8–10 blueberries 20 g walnuts	1 kiwi fruit 40–50 g casein protein 20 g walnuts	30–50 g casein protein 20 g almonds

DRINK PLENTY OF WATER! (2.5–3.5 LITRES A DAY)

Water plays an important role in lipid metabolism. It is essential for the conversion of fat into energy, reduces appetite, alleviates constipation and helps remove waste from the body, which in turn, helps keep energy levels up.

PHASE 3 SPORTS DIET WEEK 9–12

THURSDAY	FRIDAY	SATURDAY	SUNDAY	SUPPS
				(1 × daily)
omelette made with 2 whole eggs and 4–6 egg whites 1 slice toasted wholemeal bread 1 tomato	70–100 g porridge 10–12 blueberries ½ banana 30–50 g whey isolate	50–75 g cereal 20 g raisins 20 g walnuts 30–50 g whey protein	omelette made with 2 whole eggs and 4–6 egg whites 1 slice toasted wholemeal bread 1 tomato	1 BCAA multivitamin, fish oil, vitamin D
150 g chicken breast 1 green apple with cinnamon	50 g chicken breast omelette made with 3–4 egg whites 2–4 rice cakes ½ cucumber	2 slices wholemeal bread 100 g chicken breast 1 egg	150 g chicken breast 1 green apple with cinnamon	
100 g uncooked Basmati rice (cook before eating) 150 g chicken breast 150–200 g vegetables of your choice	100 g uncooked Basmati rice (cook before eating) 150 g white fish 20 g almonds 100–150 g raw vegetables	100–150 g raw vegetables ¼ avocado 150 g smoked chicken breast/salmon carpaccio	100 g uncooked Basmati rice (cook before eating) 150 g chicken breast 150–200 g vegetables of your choice	
30–50 g whey protein 2 rice cakes with peanut butter (15 g)	100 g roast beef 2–4 rice cakes 1 apple	100 g wholemeal pasta 100–150 g steak tartare tomato sauce Italian vegetable mix	30–50 g whey protein 2 rice cakes with peanut butter (15 g)	
100 g uncooked Basmati rice (cook before eating) 150 g white fish 150–200 g stir-fry vegetables 1 pineapple slice	100 g uncooked brown rice (cook before eating) 150 g chicken breast stir-fry vegetable mix 1 tablespoon olive oil	2 rice cakes 80–100 g chicken breast ½ cucumber	100 g uncooked Basmati rice (cook before eating) 150 g white fish 150–200 g stir-fry vegetables 1 pineapple slice	
250–400 g low-fat Quark 8–10 blueberries 20 g walnuts	1 kiwi fruit 40–50 g casein protein 20 g walnuts	30–50 g casein protein 20 g almonds	250–400 g low-fat Quark 8–10 blueberries 20 g walnuts	

MEN

Men who are following this plan can add 100 g meat, 100 g carbohydrates and 2 slices of wholemeal bread to the diet.

Phase 1 WEEK 1–4
DAY 1

Legs

It is important to tailor your workout to your own needs and fitness levels, so please do speak to a professional trainer before you start.

During this phase, we do 5 rounds of each of the exercises (as indicated in the green circles), interspersed with skipping. Rest for a maximum of 30 seconds between rounds. The required number of repetitions is given in the light grey boxes.

1 WARM UP

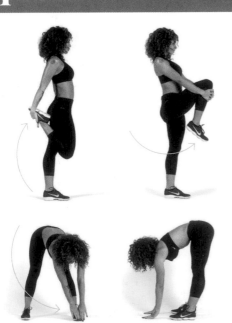

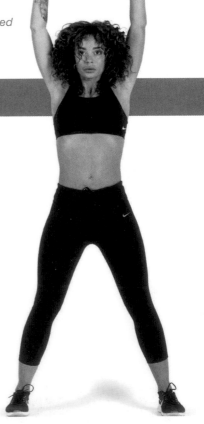

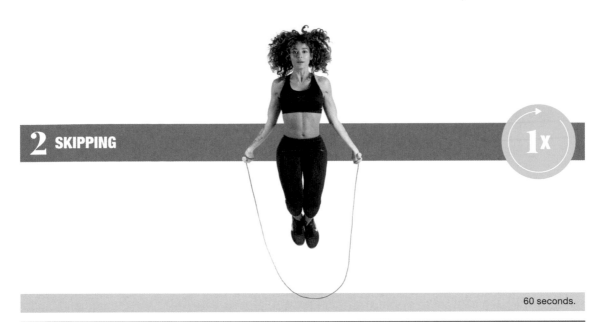

2 SKIPPING

1x

60 seconds.

3 CHAIR SQUATS

Keeping one leg lifted, lower yourself onto the chair and immediately get back up.

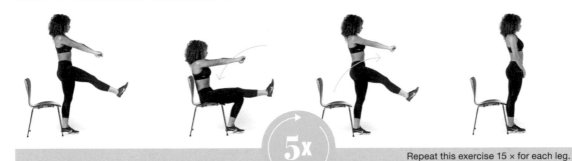

5x

Repeat this exercise 15 × for each leg.

4 FROG WALK

Crouching like a frog.

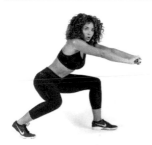

5x

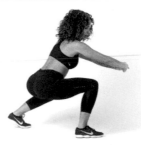

Take 10 steps forward, 10 steps back.

5 SKIPPING

1x

60 seconds.

6 SIDEWAYS WALK

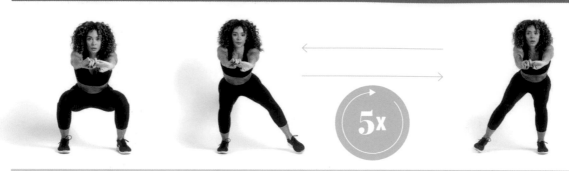

5x

15 steps to the left, 15 steps to the right.

7 SKIPPING

1x

60 seconds.

8 CRISS CROSS FLUTTER KICKS

Open and close your legs like scissors.

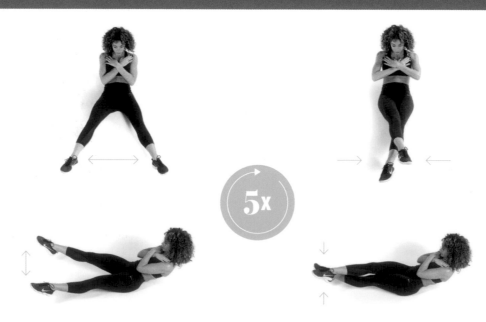

5x

30 repetitions.

9 FROG JUMPS

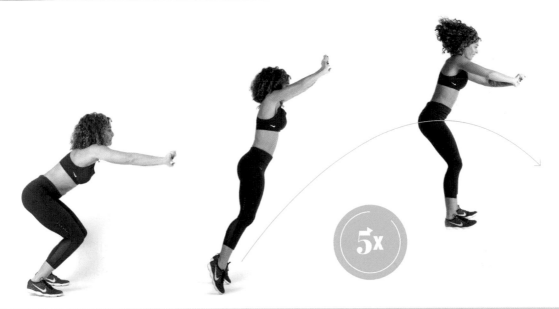

5x

15 jumps forward and 15 back.

10 SUMO SQUAT

Placing your feet a little further apart, crouch down until your knees are bent at a 90-degree angle.

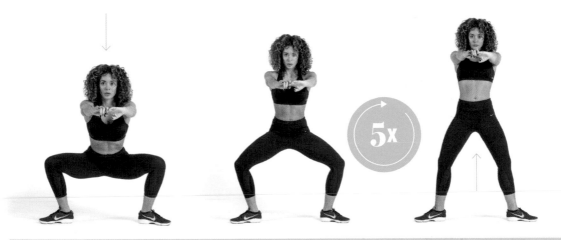

5x

15 repetitions.

Phase 1 WEEK 1–4

DAY 2

Tummy, triceps & shoulders

Start with a **WARM UP**, as on Day 1.

---

1 TRICEP DIPS　　　　　　　　　Carry on dipping until you can dip no more.

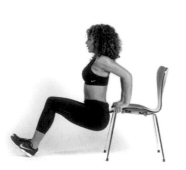
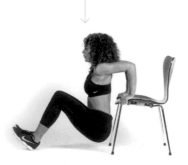
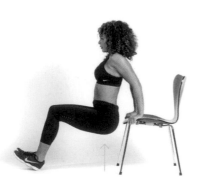
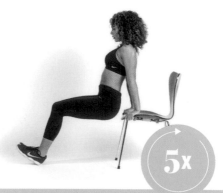

5x

Try not to count.

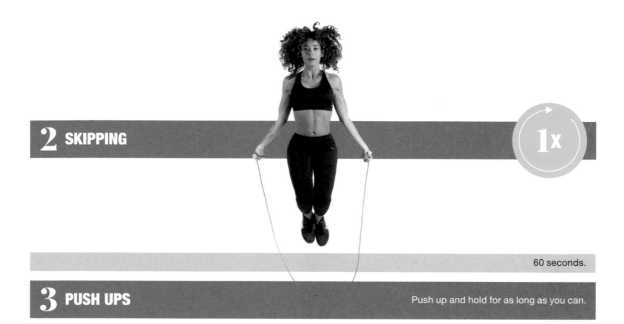

2 SKIPPING

1x

60 seconds.

3 PUSH UPS

Push up and hold for as long as you can.

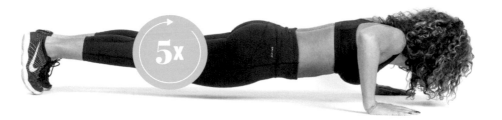

5x

Try not to count.

4 PLANK

Place elbows under shoulders and push your lower body off the floor onto your toes keeping head, neck, back and hips in a straight line, pulling in your stomach.

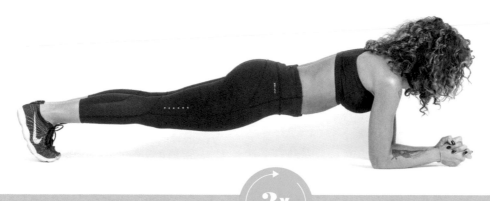

3x

30 seconds.

5 SIDE PLANK

Keep your elbow underneath the shoulder and roll onto the side of your foot. Bounce from left to right.

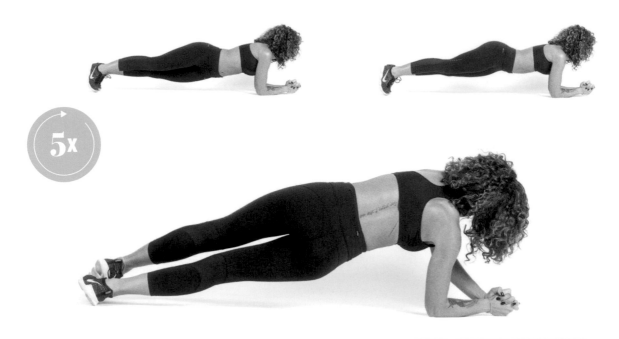

5x

15 repetitions on each side.

6 SKIPPING

1x

60 seconds.

7 SIDE RAISES USING RESISTANCE (ELASTIC) BAND OR WATER BOTTLES

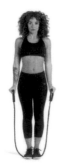
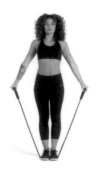
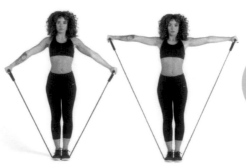
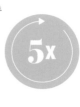

5x

15 repetitions.

8 FRONT SHOULDER FLYS

Keeping a straight back, pull in stomach muscles and raise your arms parallel to the floor.

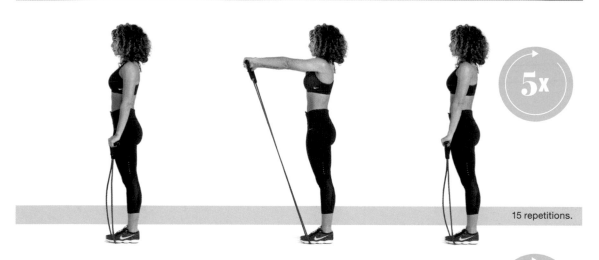

5x

15 repetitions.

9 SKIPPING

1x

60 seconds.

10 ABDOMINAL CRUNCHES

Don't strain your neck.

5x

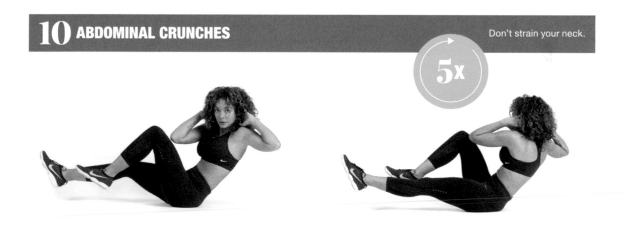

30 repetitions.

Phase 1 WEEK 1–4
DAY 3

During this phase, we do 5 rounds of each of the exercises (as indicated in the green circles), interspersed with skipping. Rest for a maximum of 30 seconds between rounds. The required number of repetitions is given in the light grey boxes.

Start with a **WARM UP** *, as on Day 1*

1 BICEP CURL USING RESISTANCE (ELASTIC) BAND

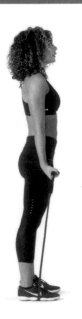
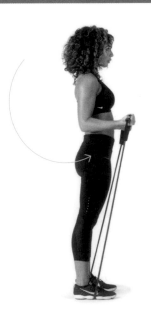

5x

15 repetitions.

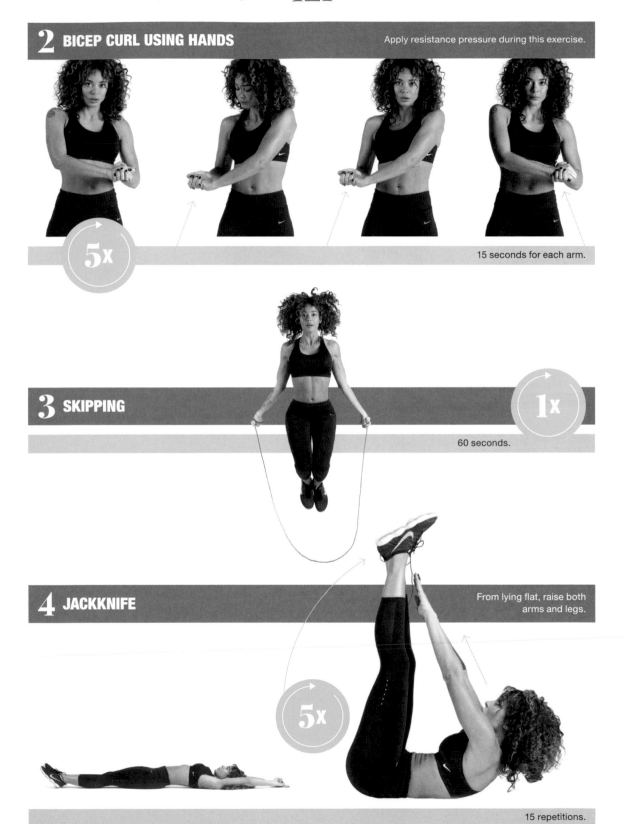

2 BICEP CURL USING HANDS

Apply resistance pressure during this exercise.

5x

15 seconds for each arm.

3 SKIPPING

1x

60 seconds.

4 JACKKNIFE

From lying flat, raise both arms and legs.

5x

15 repetitions.

5 TRAPEZE PULL

Lying on your front with chest raised, move arms front to side.

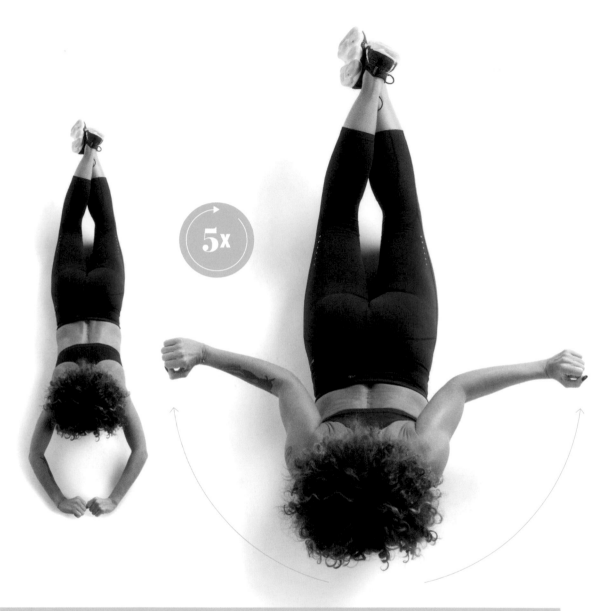

5x

15 repetitions.

6 SKIPPING

1x

60 seconds.

7 SMALL PUSH UPS

Small knee push ups; down in 3 seconds, back up in 1 second.

5x

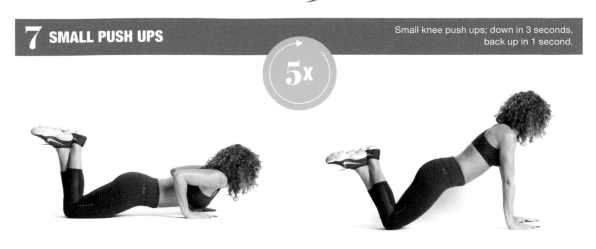

15 repetitions.

8 SKIPPING

1x

60 seconds.

9 PLANKS

3x

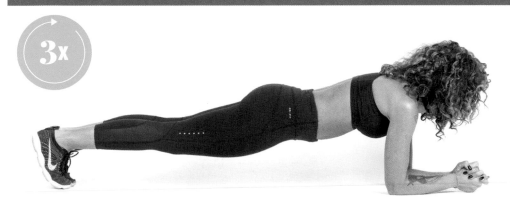

60 seconds.

Phase 2 WEEK 5–8
DAY 1

During this phase, we do the usual 5 rounds of each exercise, with 15 repetitions and a maximum of 30 seconds' rest between the exercises. The endurance exercises are now 30 seconds longer.

Start with a **WARM UP**, *as on Day 1 of Phase 1.*

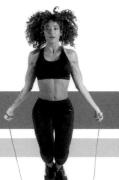

1 SKIPPING

1x

90 seconds.

2 WALKING LUNGES

15 × forward, frog jumps backwards.

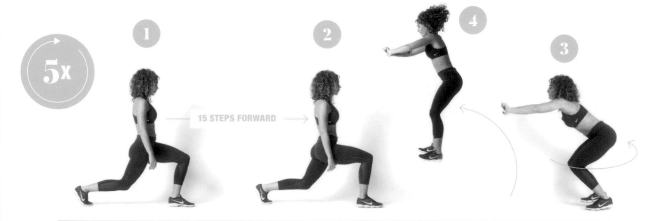

5x

1 **2** **4** **3**

15 STEPS FORWARD

15 repetitions.

3 SIDE BRIDGE

5x LEFT **5x RIGHT**

15 repetitions.

4 BURPEES

Kneel down, thrust feet back to straighten legs, push up, thrust feet forwards and jump back into standing position.

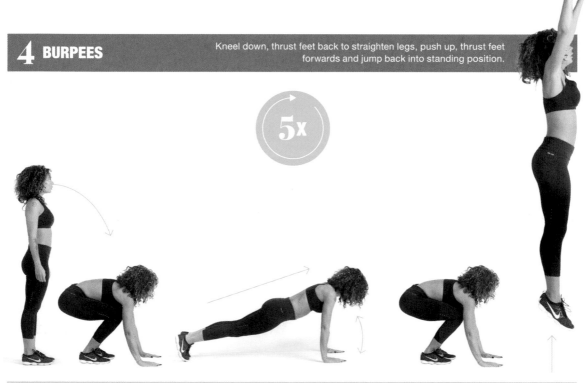

5x

15 repetitions.

5 BARBARIAN

With one foot on the chair, bend other knee until thigh is parallel to the floor; knee should not go past the foot.

5x LEFT **5x RIGHT**

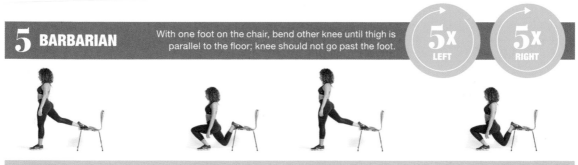

15 repetitions.

6 HIP THRUSTER

Both feet on the chair.

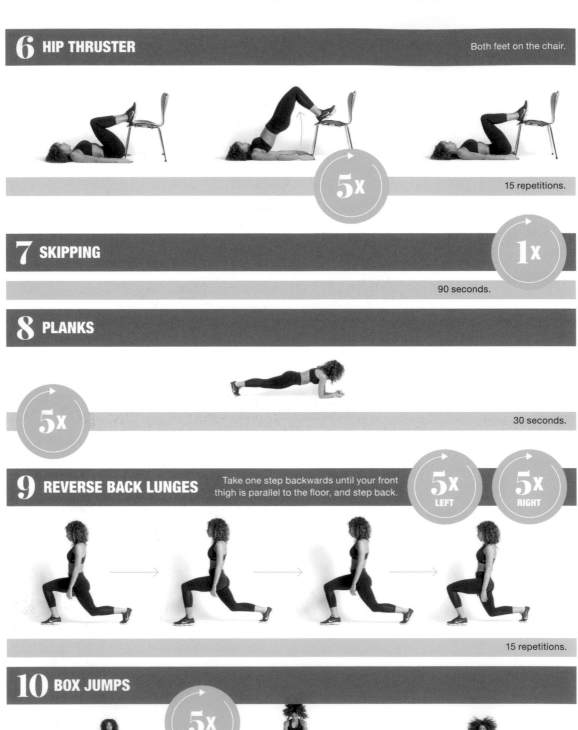

5x

15 repetitions.

7 SKIPPING

1x

90 seconds.

8 PLANKS

5x

30 seconds.

9 REVERSE BACK LUNGES

Take one step backwards until your front thigh is parallel to the floor, and step back.

5x LEFT   5x RIGHT

15 repetitions.

10 BOX JUMPS

5x

15 repetitions.

11 SWISS BALL HAMSTRING CURL

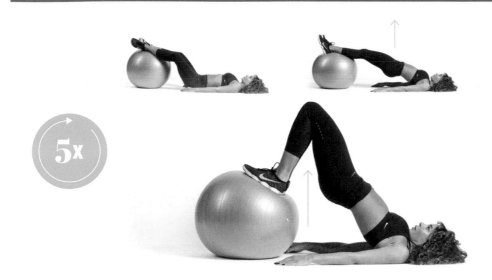

5x

15 repetitions.

12 ABDOMINAL SWISS BALL

5x

15 repetitions.

13 DONKEY KICK

On your hands and knees and looking forward, raise one leg until your thigh is parallel to the floor. Repeat with other leg.

5x

15 repetitions.

Phase 2 WEEK 5–8
DAY 2

During this phase, we do the usual 5 rounds of each exercise, with 15 repetitions and a maximum of 30 seconds' rest between the exercises. The endurance exercises are now 30 seconds longer.

Start with a **WARM UP***, as on Day 1 of Phase 1*

1 KNEE PUSH UPS   5x

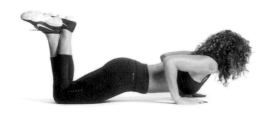

15 repetitions.

2 PLANKS

 5x

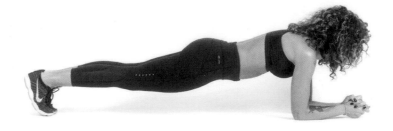

90 seconds.

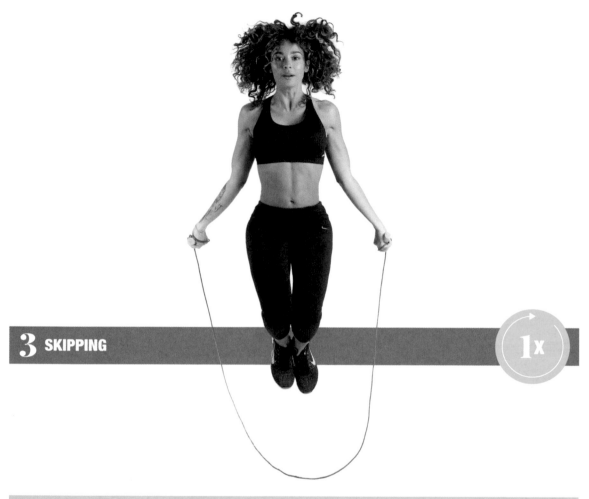

3 SKIPPING **1x**

90 seconds.

4 CRUNCHES **5x**

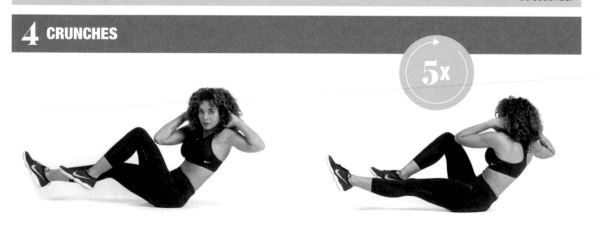

15 repetitions.

5 BURPEES

Kneel down, thrust feet back to straighten legs, push up, thrust feet forward and jump back into standing position.

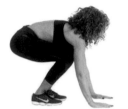
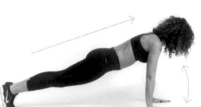
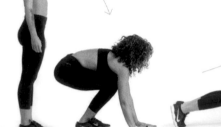

5x

15 repetitions.

6 BICEP CURL USING RESISTANCE (ELASTIC) BAND OR WATER BOTTLES

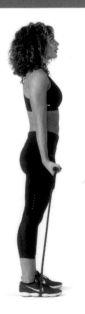
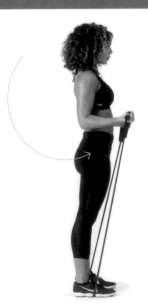

5x

15 repetitions.

7 TRICEP DIPS

Hands placed on a chair with your back close to the chair.

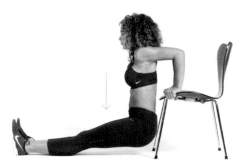

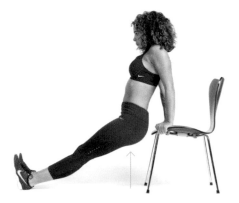

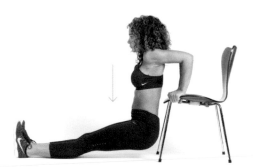

5x

15 repetitions.

Phase 2 WEEK 5–8
DAY 3

During this phase, we do the usual 5 rounds of each exercise, with 15 repetitions and a maximum of 30 seconds' rest between the exercises. The endurance exercises are now 30 seconds longer.

Start with a **WARM UP***, as on Day 1 of Phase 1*

1 SMALL ARM CIRCLES Turn small circles with your arms.

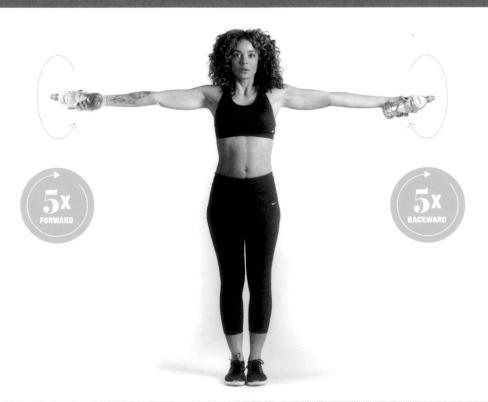

5x FORWARD

5x BACKWARD

15 repetitions.

2 SMALL ARM CIRCLES

Stretch arms out in front. Hold a bottle of water in each hand to make it harder.

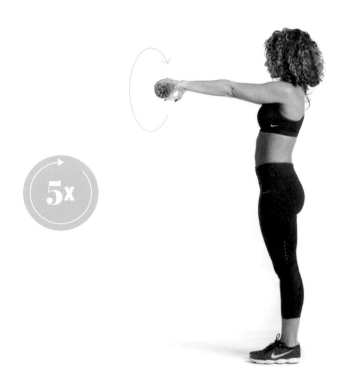

5x

15 repetitions.

3 BOXING

Holding a bottle of water in each hand.

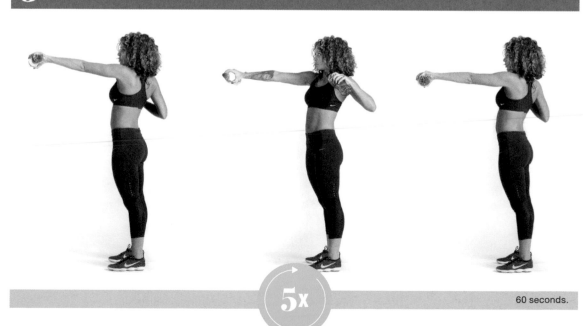

5x

60 seconds.

4 SKIPPING

1x

90 seconds.

5 PUSH UPS

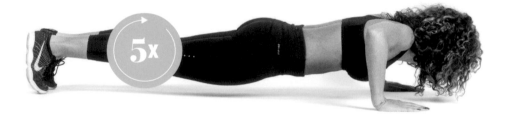

5x

15 repetitions.

6 TRAPEZIUS PULL

On the floor with a rolled-up towel.

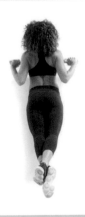
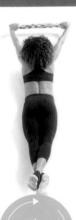
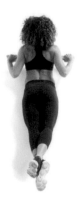

5x

15 repetitions.

7 COBRA

Lying on your front, raise your upper body and thighs.

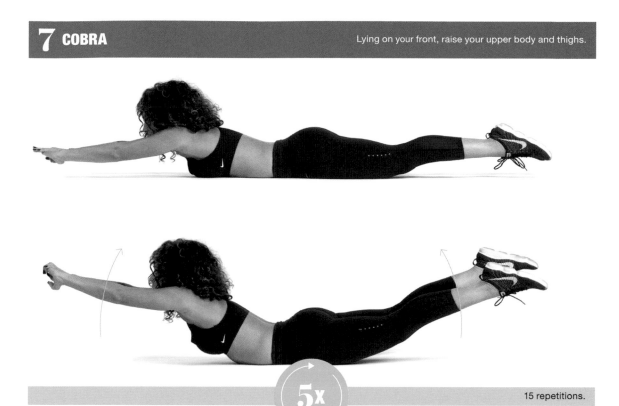

5x

15 repetitions.

8 SKIPPING

1x

90 seconds.

Phase 3 WEEK 9–12
DAY 1

During this phase, we do 10 × 10 'supersets', meaning we do 2 exercises in succession, followed by 30 seconds' rest. You do 10 rounds, each with 10 repetitions; there are not as many different exercises, but more rounds.

Start with a **WARM UP***, as on Day 1 of Phase 1*

1 SUMO SQUAT

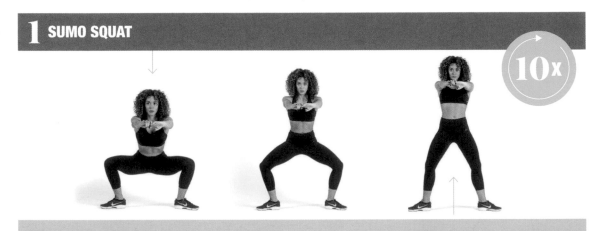

10x

+

2 SQUATS

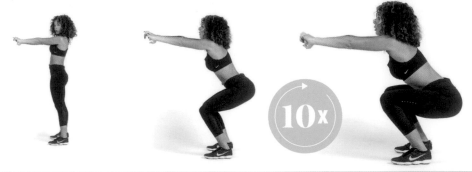

10x

Repeat these 2 exercises 10 times.

3 ONE LEG BARBARIAN SQUAT

Keeping one leg raised, lower yourself down onto the chair and back up.

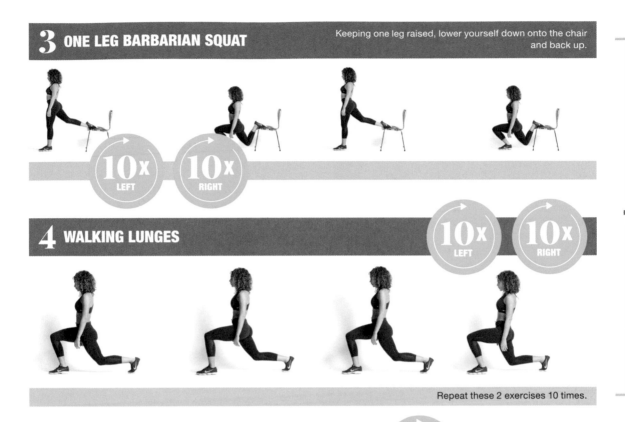

10x LEFT **10x RIGHT**

4 WALKING LUNGES

10x LEFT **10x RIGHT**

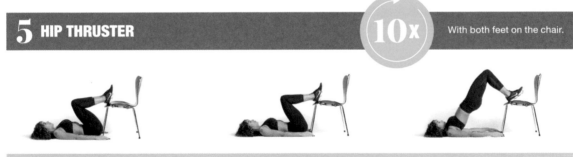

Repeat these 2 exercises 10 times.

5 HIP THRUSTER

10x With both feet on the chair.

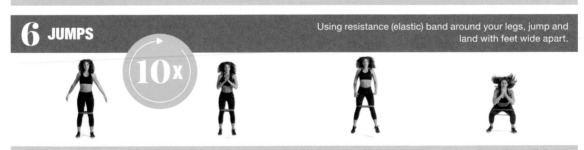

6 JUMPS

Using resistance (elastic) band around your legs, jump and land with feet wide apart.

10x

Repeat these 2 exercises 10 times.

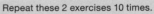

Phase 3 WEEK 9–12
DAY 2

During this phase, we do 10 × 10 'supersets', meaning we do 2 exercises in succession, followed by 30 seconds' rest. You do 10 rounds, each with 10 repetitions; there are not as many different exercises, but more rounds.

Start with a **WARM UP***, as on Day 1 of Phase 1*

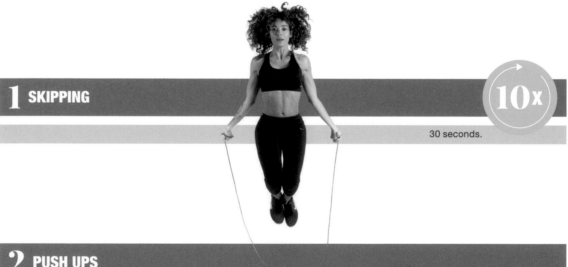

1 SKIPPING 10x 30 seconds.

2 PUSH UPS 10x

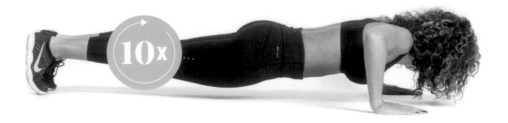

Repeat these 2 exercises 10 times.

3 TRICEPS ON A CHAIR OR SWISS BALL

10x

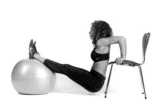
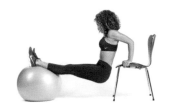
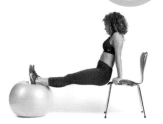

4 TRICEPS PUSH UPS

Hands not too far apart, keeping arms close to your body.

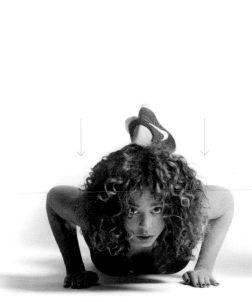
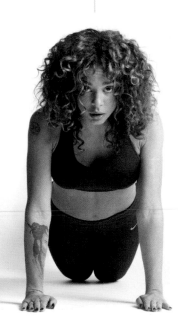

10x

Repeat these 2 exercises 10 times.

5 PLANKS

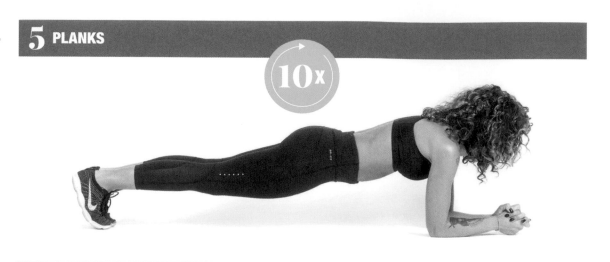

60 seconds.

6 COBRA

Raise both arms and legs at the same time.

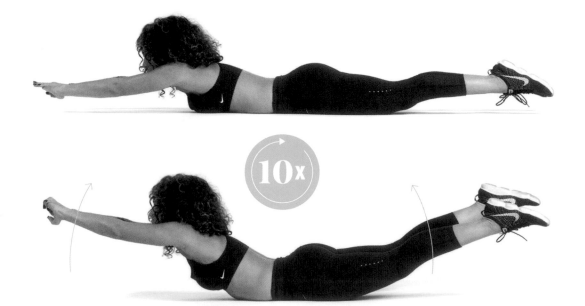

Repeat these 2 exercises 10 times.

7 TRAPEZIUS PULL

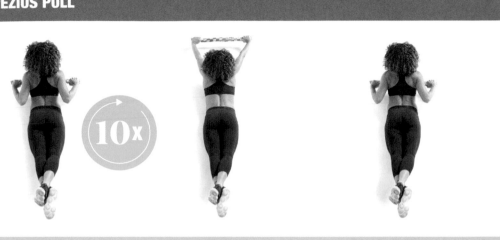

10x

8 SKIPPING

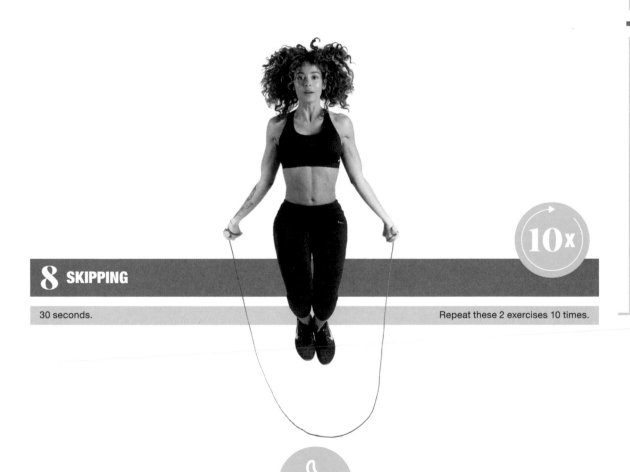

10x

30 seconds.

Repeat these 2 exercises 10 times.

Phase 3 WEEK 9–12
DAY 3

During this phase, we do 10 × 10 'supersets', meaning we do two exercises in succession, followed by 30 seconds' rest. You do 10 rounds, each with 10 repetitions; there are not as many different exercises, but more rounds.

Start with a **WARM UP***, as on Day 1 of Phase 1*

1 SPIDERMAN PUSH UPS   From a push up position, bring your right knee to your right elbow.

10x EACH LEG

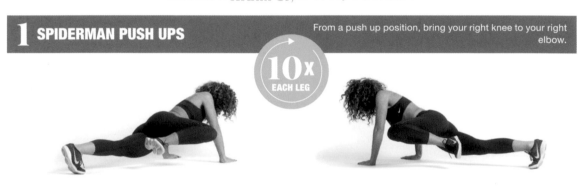

10x

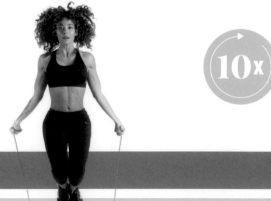

2 SKIPPING

30 seconds.   Repeat these 2 exercises 10 times.

3 PLANKS

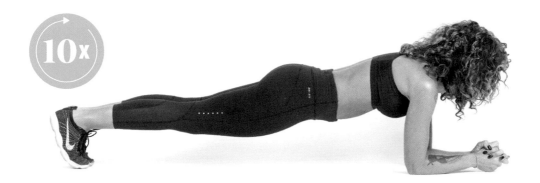

10x

30 seconds.

4 SIDE PLANK

Keep elbows underneath your shoulders and roll onto the side of your foot. Bounce from left to right.

10x

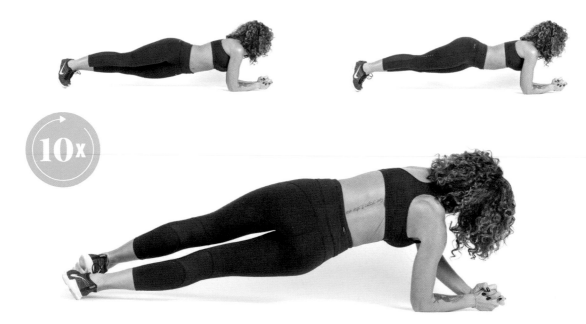

Repeat these 2 exercises 10 times.

5 BICEP CURL USING RESISTANCE (ELASTIC) BAND

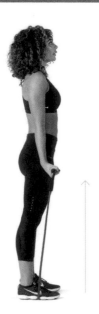
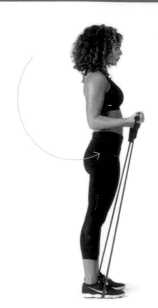

6 BURPEES

Kneel down, thrust feet back to straighten your legs, push up, thrust feet forward and jump back into standing position.

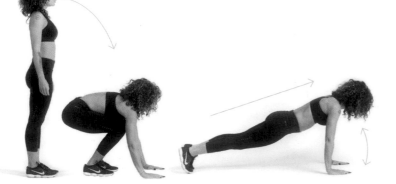
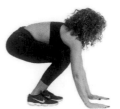

Repeat these 2 exercises 10 times.

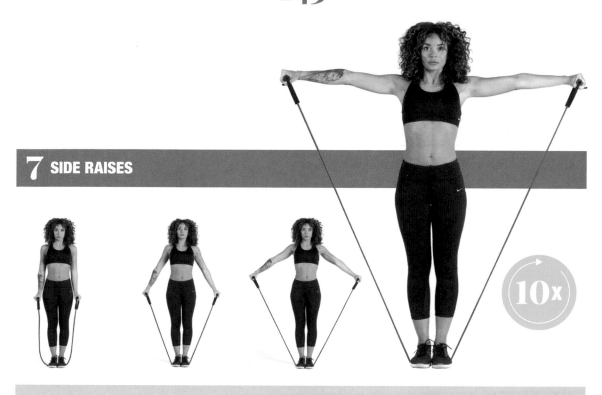

7 SIDE RAISES

10x

8 FRONT RAISES

10x

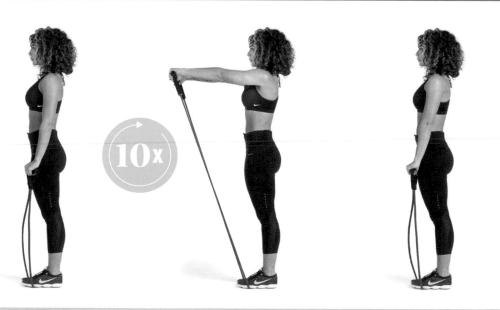

Repeat these 2 exercises 10 times.

9 SKIPPING

10x

30 seconds.

10 CRUNCHES

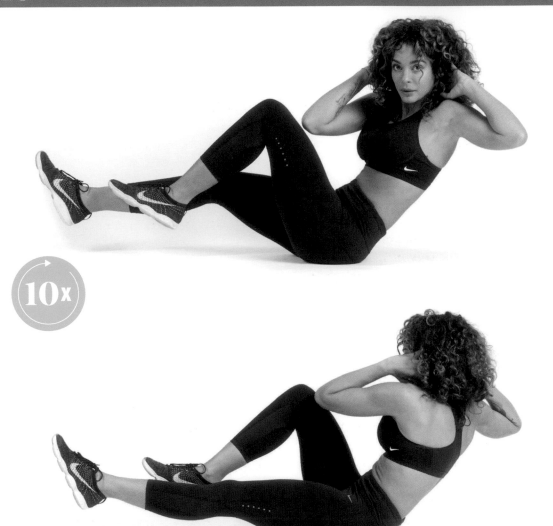

10x

30 seconds.

Repeat these 2 exercises 10 times.

Effective training: variation and focus

You can make your training (even more) effective by paying attention to 2 key aspects: variation and focus – and particularly the combination of these 2.

Variation probably speaks for itself: if you stick to the same regime for too, long your body will get bored with it. But you can avoid this by changing your exercise routine regularly and pushing yourself to make it harder as you progress: keep increasing the number of repetitions as well as the weights you use.

Focus relates to the actual objective of your training – is it muscle growth or getting leaner? It's true that the same exercises can probably suit both but what matters is how you do them. If your aim is more muscle, you should go for heavy weights but fewer repetitions. Getting leaner can, on the other hand, be achieved by more repetitions (12–18 times) and adding a lot of plyometric exercises (fast, powerful and explosive movements) and HIIT (High Intensity Interval Training) to your workout. Ask someone at the gym about this.

To illustrate, doing squats can serve both purposes: muscle growth and getting lean. However, if the focus is on muscle growth, you might do 6 sets of 6 repetitions using heavy weights and taking at least 60 seconds'

rest between sets. If the objective is to get leaner, you would do only 4 sets, going up to perhaps 18 repetitions using lighter weights and only 30 seconds' rest between sets.

'TOP TIP: ALTERNATE BETWEEN THE 2 OBJECTIVES'

Bearing in mind the need to vary your training depending on what you are focusing on, here is a top tip: alternate between the 2 objectives. In other words: variation in focus is key to getting the most out of your training in terms of muscle growth and physical development. By frequently changing your workouts, your body will be stimulated and stretched by the unfamiliar – especially if you use much heavier weights when doing sets with fewer repetitions because, even though you are not moving as much, each movement will take a lot more effort and place different demands on your muscles.

However, rather than randomly mixing up all the different training methods, take a structured approach otherwise your body will get confused, which may actually hamper

Phase 1 WEEK 1–4
2 DAYS' TRAINING

In Phase 1, you are aiming high: 15–18 repetitions, struggling to finish the exercise by the time you reach 16.

DAY 1 *Biceps, triceps & chest*

1 **FLAT DUMBBELL PRESS – PUSH UPS** 5 rounds — 15-18x

2 **ALTERNATE STANDING DUMBBELL CURL** 5 rounds — 15-18x

3 **CABLE ROPE PUSH DOWN** 5 rounds — 15-18x

4 **SEATED MACHINE PRESS** 5 rounds — 15-18x

5 **SIDE LATERAL RAISES** 5 rounds — 15-18x

6 **OVERHAND WIDE GRIP LAT PULL DOWNS** 5 rounds — 15-18x

7 **SEATED ROWS (CLOSE GRIP)** 5 rounds — 15-18x

8 **LEG EXTENSIONS** 5 rounds — 15-18x

9 **HAMSTRING CURLS** 5 rounds — 15-18x

DAY 2 *Quadriceps, hamstrings & calves*

1 **SMITH MACHINE SQUATS** 5 rounds — 15-18x

2 **WALKING LUNGES** 5 rounds — 15-18x

3 **STIFF LEGGED DEADLIFTS** 5 rounds — 15-18x

4 **UNDERHAND GRIP BARBELL ROWS** 5 rounds — 15-18x

5 **LOW PULLEY CABLES TO FRONT RAISE (CABLE MACHINE)** 5 rounds — 15-18x

6 **SEATED DUMBBELL PRESS** 5 rounds — 15-18x

7 **INCLINE DUMBBELL CURL** 5 rounds — 15-18x

8 **STRAIGHT BAR PRESS DOWN** 5 rounds — 15-18x

Phase 2 WEEK 5–8
2 DAYS' TRAINNG

During Phase 2, you do a set of 3 exercises in succession, taking 60 seconds' rest after the third exercise. You do 8 repetitions of the first exercise, 12 of the second and 25 repetitions of the third. Repeat this sequence 5 times.

DAY 1 *Total body*

1 **CABLE CROSS OVERS** — 8x

2 **CABLE CURLS** — 12x

3 **ROPE OVER HEAD EXTENSION** 5 sets, 60 seconds' rest after each set — 25x

4 **SIDE LATERAL RAISES** — 8x

5 **UP RIGHT ROWS** — 12x

6 **UNDERHAND GRIP BARBELL ROWS** 5 sets, 60 seconds' rest after each set — 25x

7 **HYPEREXTENSION** — 8x

8 BARBELL SQUAT `12x`

9 SEATED LEG CURL `25x`
5 sets, 60 seconds' rest after each set

DAY 2 *Total body*

1 LEG PRESS `8x`

2 LEG EXTENSIONS `12x`

3 SEATED LEG CURL `25x`
5 sets, 60 seconds' rest after each set

4 REVERSE GRIP PULL DOWN `8x`

5 DUMBBELL FRONT RAISES `12x`

6 SEATED DUMBBELL PRESS `25x`
5 sets, 60 seconds' rest after each set

7 STANDING BARBELL CURL `8x`

8 DUMBBELL KICKBACK each arm `12x`

9 TRICEP DIPS `25x`
5 sets, 60 seconds' rest after each set

Phase 3 WEEK 9–12
2 DAYS' TRAINING
Supersets: 6 repetitions, as demanding as possible.

DAY 1 *Biceps, triceps & chest*

1 INCLINE DUMBBELL PRESS `6x`

2 SEATED INCLINE DUMBBELL CURL `6x`
5 sets, 60 seconds' rest after each set

3 SEATED DUMBBELL EXTENSION `6x`

4 SEATED DUMBBELL PRESS `6x`
5 sets, 60 seconds' rest after each set

5 CABLE SIDE LATERAL RAISES `6x`

6 SEATED CABLE ROW `6x`
5 sets, 60 seconds' rest after each set

7 REVERSE GRIP LAT PULL DOWN `6x`

8 LEG EXTENSIONS `6x`
5 sets, 60 seconds' rest after each set

DAY 2 *Quadriceps & hamstrings*

1 BARBELL SQUAT `6x`

2 SMITH MACHINE LUNGES `6x`
5 sets, 60 seconds' rest after each set

3 LYING OR SEATED LEG CURL `6x`

4 ONE-ARM DUMBBELL ROW `6x`
5 sets, 60 seconds' rest after each set

5 LAT PULL DOWN FRONT AND REAR `6x`

6 MACHINE SHOULDER PRESS `6x`
5 sets, 60 seconds' rest after each set

7 STANDING BAR CURLS `6x`

8 STRAIGHT BAR PRESS DOWN `8x`
5 sets, 60 seconds' rest after each set

Phase 1 WEEK 1–4
3 DAYS' TRAINING

In Phase 1, you are aiming high: 15–18 repetitions, struggling to finish by the time you reach 16.

DAY 2 *Quadriceps, hamstrings & calves*

1	**LEG EXTENSIONS** 5 rounds	15–18x
2	**LEG PRESS** 5 rounds	15–18x
3	**WALKING LUNGES** 5 rounds	15–18x
4	**HAMSTRING CURLS** 5 rounds	15–18x
5	**SUMO SMITH MACHINE SQUATS** 5 rounds	15–18x
6	**STIFF-LEGGED DEADLIFTS** 5 rounds	15–18x
7	**STANDING CALF RAISES** 5 rounds	15–18x
8	**SEATED CALF RAISES** 5 rounds	15–18x

DAY 1 *Biceps, triceps & chest*

1	**INCLINE BARBELL PRESS** 5 rounds	15–18x
2	**FLAT DUMBBELL PRESS PUSH UPS** 5 rounds	15–18x
3	**CABLE CROSS OVERS** 5 rounds	15–18x
4	**STANDING ALTERNATE DUMBBELL CURL** 5 rounds	15–18x
5	**BICEP CABLE CURLS** 5 rounds	15–18x
6	**V-BAR PUSH DOWNS** 5 rounds	15–18x
7	**CABLE ROPE PUSH DOWNS** 5 rounds	15–18x

DAY 3 *Shoulders & back*

1	**STRAIGHT ARM ROPE PULL DOWNS** 5 rounds	15–18x
2	**OVERHAND WIDE GRIP LAT PULL DOWNS** 5 rounds	15–18x
3	**UNDER HAND GRIP BARBELL ROWS** 5 rounds	15–18x
4	**SEATED ROWS (CLOSE GRIP)** 5 rounds	15–18x
5	**SEATED MACHINE PRESS** 5 rounds	15–18x
6	**LOW PULLEY CABLES TO FRONT RAISE (CABLE MACHINE)** 5 rounds	15–18x
7	**SIDE LATERAL RAISES** 5 rounds	15–18x

Phase 2 WEEK 5–8
3 DAYS' TRAINING

During Phase 2, you do a set of 3 exercises in succession, taking 60 seconds' rest after the third exercise. You do 8 repetitions of the first exercise, 12 of the second and 25 repetitions of the third. Repeat this sequence 5 times.

DAY 1 *Biceps, triceps & chest*

1	CABLE CROSS OVERS	8x
2	INCLINE SMITH MACHINE PRESS	12x
3	INCLINE FLYS 5 sets, 60 seconds' rest after each set	25x
4	STRAIGHT BARBELL CURLS	8x
5	CABLE CURLS	12x
6	ROPE OVERHEAD EXTENSION 5 sets, 60 seconds' rest after each set	25x
7	DUMBBELL KICKBACK each arm	8x
8	DUMBBELL BICEP CURLS	25x
9	ONE ARM DUMBBELL PRESS each arm 5 sets, 60 seconds' rest after each set	12x

DAY 2 *Quadriceps, hamstrings & calves*

1	LEG EXTENSIONS	8x
2	SQUAT	12x
3	LEG PRESS 5 sets, 60 seconds' rest after each set	25x
4	ABDUCTOR MACHINE	8x
5	STIFF-LEGGED DEADLIFTS	12x
6	SEATED LEG CURL 5 sets, 60 seconds' rest after each set	25x
7	LYING LEG CURL	8x
8	SEATED CALF RAISES	12x
9	FROG JUMPS 5 sets, 60 seconds' rest after each set	25x

DAY 3 *Shoulders & back*

1	UNDERHAND GRIP BARBELL ROWS	8x
2	OVERHAND GRIP LAT PULL DOWNS – LEANING RIGHT BACK FRONT LAT PULL DOWNS	12x
3	HYPEREXTENSIONS 5 sets, 60 seconds' rest after each set	25x
4	SEATED MACHINE PRESS – SIDE LATERAL RAISES	8x
5	UPRIGHT ROWS	12x
6	UNDERHAND GRIP FRONT RAISE 5 sets, 60 seconds' rest after each set	25x
7	PULL UPS	8x
8	BENT-OVER RAISES	12x
9	SHOULDER PRESS 5 sets, 60 seconds' rest after each set	25x

Phase 3 WEEK 9–12
3 DAYS' TRAINING

In Phase 3, you step up the pace with supersets, each consisting of 2 exercises repeated 6 times, making them as demanding as possible. Every set is repeated 5 times.

DAY 2 *Quadriceps, hamstrings & calves*

1 **LEG PRESS** 6x

2 **SMITH MACHINE SQUATS**
5 sets, 60 seconds' rest after each set 6x

3 **STEP-UPS (BLOCK OR BENCH)** 6x

4 **LEG EXTENSIONS**
5 sets, 60 seconds' rest after each set 6x

5 **LYING LEG CURL** 6x

6 **LUNGES**
5 sets, 60 seconds' rest after each set 6x

7 **SEATED LEG CURL** 6x

8 **STANDING CALF RAISES**
5 sets, 60 seconds' rest after each set 6x

DAY 1 *Biceps, triceps & chest*

1 **DIPS** With your feet on the bench and a 5-kilo weight on your legs 6x

2 **BENCH PRESS**
5 sets, 60 seconds' rest after each set 6x

3 **FLAT SMITH MACHINE PRESS** 6x

4 **PUSH UPS**
5 sets, 60 seconds' rest after each set 6x

5 **SEATED DUMBBELL CURL** 6x

6 **CABLE CURLS**
5 sets, 60 seconds' rest after each set 6x

7 **SEATED DUMBBELL EXTENSION** 6x

8 **V-BAR PUSH DOWNS**
5 sets, 60 seconds' rest after each set 6x

DAY 3 *Shoulders & back*

1 **REVERSE GRIP FRONT LAT PULL DOWN** 6x

2 **OVERHAND GRIP BARBELL**
5 sets, 60 seconds' rest after each set 6x

3 **SEATED CABLE ROW** 6x

4 **ONE-ARM DUMBBELL ROW**
5 sets, 60 seconds' rest after each set 6x

5 **BAR FRONT RAISES** 6x

6 **REAR CABLE DELT**
5 sets, 60 seconds' rest after each set 6x

7 **DUMBBELL PRESS** 6x

8 **PULL UPS** 8x

Phase 1 WEEK 1–4
4 DAYS' TRAINING

In Phase 1, you are aiming high: 15–18 repetitions, struggling to finish by the time you get to 16.

DAY 1 *Biceps & chest*

1. **INCLINE BARBELL PRESS** 5 rounds — 15-18x
2. **SEATED MACHINE PRESS** 5 rounds — 15-18x
3. **FLAT DUMBBELL PRESS PUSH UP** 5 rounds — 15-18x
4. **CABLE CROSS OVERS** 5 rounds — 15-18x
5. **ALTERNATE STANDING DUMBBELL CURL** 5 rounds — 15-18x
6. **BICEP CABLE CURLS** 5 rounds — 15-18x

DAY 2 *Quadriceps & hamstrings*

1. **LEG EXTENSIONS** 5 rounds — 15-18x
2. **LEG PRESS** 5 rounds — 15-18x
3. **LEG EXTENSION – WALKING LUNGES** 5 rounds — 15-18x
4. **HAMSTRING CURLS** 5 rounds — 15-18x
5. **SUMO SMITH MACHINE SQUATS** 5 rounds — 15-18x
6. **STIFF-LEGGED DEADLIFTS** 5 rounds — 15-18x

DAY 3 *Back & calves*

1. **STRAIGHT-ARM ROPE PULL DOWNS** 5 rounds — 15-18x
2. **OVERHAND WIDE GRIP LAT PULL DOWNS** 5 rounds — 15-18x
3. **UNDERHAND GRIP BARBELL ROWS** 5 rounds — 15-18x
4. **SEATED ROWS (CLOSE GRIP)** 5 rounds — 15-18x
5. **STANDING CALF RAISES** 5 rounds — 15-18x
6. **SEATED CALF RAISES** 5 rounds — 15-18x

DAY 4 *Deltoids* & triceps*

1. **SINGLE ARM LAT RAISES** (lying on an incline bench) 5 rounds — 15-18x
2. **SEATED MACHINE PRESS** 5 rounds — 15-18x
3. **LOW-PULLEY CABLES TO FRONT RAISE (CABLE MACHINE)** 5 rounds — 15-18x
4. **SIDE LATERAL RAISES** 5 rounds — 15-18x
5. **REVERSE GRIP PUSH DOWNS** 5 rounds — 15-18x
6. **V-BAR PUSH DOWNS** 5 rounds — 15-18x
7. **CABLE ROPE PUSH DOWNS** 5 rounds — 15-18x

* The deltoid muscle is located between the trapezius and biceps and upper arm, and enables the arm to lift and turn.

Phase 2 WEEK 5–8
4 DAYS' TRAINING

During Phase 2, we will do a set of 3 exercises in succession, taking 60 seconds' rest after the third exercise. You do 8 repetitions of the first exercise, 12 of the second and 25 repetitions of the third. Repeat this sequence 5 times.

DAY 1 *Biceps, triceps & chest*

1	CABLE CROSS OVERS	8x
2	SEATED MACHINE PRESS	12x
3	INCLINE FLYS 5 sets, 60 seconds' rest after each set	25x
4	INCLINE SMITH MACHINE PRESS	8x
5	STRAIGHT BARBELL CURLS	12x
6	CABLE CURLS 5 sets, 60 seconds' rest after each set	25x

DAY 2 *Quadriceps & hamstrings*

1	LEG PRESS	8x
2	SQUATS	12x
3	LEG EXTENSIONS 5 sets, 60 seconds' rest after each set	25x
4	STIFF-LEGGED DEADLIFTS	8x
5	SEATED LEG CURL	12x
6	HAMSTRING CURL 5 sets, 60 seconds' rest after each set	25x

DAY 3 *Back*

1	STRAIGHT-ARM ROPE PULL DOWNS	8x
2	UNDERHAND GRIP BARBELL ROWS	12x
3	OVERHAND GRIP LAT PULL DOWNS – SS LEANING RIGHT 5 sets, 60 seconds' rest after each set	25x
4	HYPEREXTENSTION	8x
5	STANDING CALF RAISES	12x
6	SEATED CALF RAISES 5 sets, 60 seconds' rest after each set	25x

DAY 4 *Deltoids & triceps*

1	SIDE LATERAL RAISES	8x
2	SEATED MACHINE PRESS – SIDE LATERAL RAISES	12x
3	UPRIGHT ROWS 5 sets, 60 seconds' rest after each set	25x
4	DUMBBELL KICKBACK	8x
5	ROPE OVERHEAD EXTENSION	12x
6	UNDERHAND GRIP FRONT RAISE 5 sets, 60 seconds' rest after each set	25x

Phase 3 WEEK 9–12
4 DAYS TRAINING

Supersets: 6 repetitions, as demanding as possible!

DAY 1 *Chest*

1	INCLINE FLYS	6x
2	BENCH PRESS *5 sets, 60 seconds' rest after each set*	6x
3	FLAT SMITH MACHINE PRESS	6x
4	PUSH UPS *5 sets, 60 seconds' rest after each set*	6x
5	SEATED DUMBBELL CURL	6x
6	CABLE CURLS *5 sets, 60 seconds' rest after each set*	6x
7	PREACHER CURLS	6x
8	PUSH UPS *5 sets, 60 seconds' rest after each set*	6x

DAY 2 *Quadriceps*

1	LEG PRESS SINGLE LEG	6x
2	SQUATS *5 sets, 60 seconds' rest after each set*	6x
3	STEP-UPS (BLOCK OR BENCH)	6x
4	LEG EXTENSIONS *5 sets, 60 seconds' rest after each set*	6x
5	HAMSTRING CURL	6x
6	DUMBBELL SUMO SQUAT *5 sets, 60 seconds' rest after each set*	6x
7	LUNGES	6x
8	FROG JUMPS *5 sets, 60 seconds' rest after each set*	6x

DAY 3 *Back*

1	REVERSE GRIP FRONT LAT PULL DOWN	6x
2	OVERHAND GRIP BARBELL ROWS WIDE GRIP *5 sets, 60 seconds' rest after each set*	6x
3	SEATED CABLE ROW	6x
4	ONE ARM DUMBBELL ROW *5 sets, 60 seconds' rest after each set*	6x
5	PULL-OVER DUMBBELL	6x
6	STANDING CALF RAISES *5 sets, 60 seconds' rest after each set*	6x
7	SEATED CALF RAISES	6x
8	STRAIGHT BAR PUSH DOWN *3 × 10 min, 2 drops*	6x

DAY 4 *Deltoids*

1	SIDE LATERAL RAISES	6x
2	BAR FRONT RAISES *5 sets, 60 seconds' rest after each set*	6x
3	REAR CABLE DELT	6x
4	DUMBBELL PRESS *5 sets, 60 seconds' rest after each set*	6x
5	SEATED DUMBBELL EXTENSION	6x
6	REVERSE GRIP PUSH DOWNS *5 sets, 60 seconds' rest after each set*	6x
7	V-BAR PUSH DOWNS	6x
8	SHOULDER PRESS *5 sets, 60 seconds' rest after each set*	6x

Phase 1 WEEK 1–4
5 DAYS' TRAINING

In Phase 1, you are aiming high: 15–18 repetitions, struggling to finish by the time you get to 16.

DAY 1 *Biceps & glutes*

1	**BICEPS CABLE CURLS** 5 rounds	15-18x
2	**DUMBBELL BICEPS CURL** 5 rounds	15-18x
3	**BARBELL PREACHER CURL** 5 rounds	15-18x
4	**PUSH UPS** 5 rounds	15-18x
5	**FROG JUMPS** 5 rounds	15-18x
6	**WALL SIT** 5 rounds	15-18x
7	**SMITH MACHINE DONKEY KICKS** 5 rounds	15-18x
8	**SMITH MACHINE SUMO SQUAT** 5 rounds	15-18x
9	**SMITH MACHINE LEG PRESS** 5 rounds	15-18x
10	**WALKING LUNGES** 5 rounds	15-18x
11	**HAMSTRING CURL** 5 rounds	15-18x

DAY 2 *Triceps & chest*

1	**INCLINE BARBELL PRESS** 5 rounds	15-18x
2	**FLAT DUMBBELL PRESS PUSH UPS** 5 rounds	15-18x
3	**INCLINE SMITH MACHINE PRESS** 5 rounds	15-18x
4	**CABLE CROSS OVER** (Keep hands high, level with upper chest), 5 rounds	15-18x
5	**DIPS** 5 rounds	15-18x
6	**LYING BARBELL TRICEPS EXTENSION** 5 rounds	15-18x
7	**TRICEPS CABLE PUSH DOWN** 5 rounds	15-18x
8	**TRICEPS KICKBACK** 5 rounds	15-18x

DAY 4 *Back*

1	**PULL UPS** 5 rounds	15-18x
2	**STRAIGHT ARM ROPE PULL DOWNS** 5 rounds	15-18x
3	**WIDE GRIP LAT PULL DOWNS** 5 rounds	15-18x
4	**UNDERHAND GRIP BARBELL ROWS** 5 rounds	15-18x
5	**SEATED ROW (CLOSE GRIP)** 5 rounds	15-18x
6	**PARTIAL DEADLIFTS** 5 rounds	15-18x
7	20 min. walking on treadmill at speed 90/110	

DAY 3 *Legs*

1	**SQUAT** 5 rounds	15-18x
2	**LEG PRESS** 5 rounds	15-18x
3	**ONE LEG SQUAT** 5 rounds	15-18x
4	**WALL SIT** 3 × 45 seconds	
5	**BARBELL STIFF-LEGGED DEADLIFTS** 5 rounds	15-18x
6	**SMITH MACHINE STANDING CALF RAISES** 5 rounds	15-18x
7	**HAMSTRING CURLS** 5 rounds	15-18x
8	**LEG EXTENSION** 5 rounds	15-18x

DAY 5 *Shoulders*

1	**SHOULDER PRESS** 5 rounds	15-18x
2	**ARNOLD PRESS** 5 rounds	15-18x
3	**FRONT RAISES** (both arms at once), 5 rounds	15-18x
4	**SIDE RAISES** 5 rounds	15-18x
5	**UPRIGHT ROWS** 5 rounds	15-18x
6	20 min. walking on incline treadmill	

Phase 2 WEEK 5–8
5 DAYS' TRAINING

During Phase 2, we will do a set of 3 exercises in succession, taking 60 seconds' rest after the third exercise. You do 8 repetitions of the first exercise, 12 of the second and 25 repetitions of the third. Repeat this sequence 5 times.

DAY 1 *Biceps & glutes*

1 STANDING DUMBBELL BICEPS CURL	8x
2 HAMMER CURL	12x
3 BICEPS CURL PULLEY 5 sets, 60 seconds' rest after each set	25x
4 HIP THRUSTER	8x
5 KETTLEBELL SUMO SQUAT	12x
6 SWISS BALL HAMSTRING CURL 5 sets, with 60 seconds' rest after each set	25x

DAY 2 *Triceps & chest*

1 TRICEPS KICKBACK each arm	8x
2 TRICEPS DIPS feet on bench	12x
3 TRICEPS ROPE PUSH DOWN 5 sets, 60 seconds' rest after each set	25x
4 INCLINE FLYS	8x
5 CABLE CROSS OVERS	12x
6 SEATED MACHINE PRESS 5 sets, 60 seconds' rest after each set	25x

DAY 3 *Legs*

1 SQUAT	8x
2 FROG JUMPS	12x
3 WALKING LUNGES each leg 5 sets, 60 seconds' rest after each set	25x
4 ONE-LEG HAMSTRING CURL each leg	8x
5 ONE-LEG LEG PRESS each leg (foot against upper edge of pad)	12x
6 LEG EXTENSION 5 sets, 60 seconds' rest after each set	25x
7 STANDING CALF RAISES 3 rounds 5 sets, 60 seconds' rest after each set	30x
8 10x 10 sec. 'deadmill sprints' i.e. running on turned-off treadmill so you power the belt with your own legs. After 10 seconds, take 10 seconds' rest and so on.	

DAY 4 *Back*

1	**PULL UPS**	8x
2	**ONE-ARM ROW**	12x
3	**STRAIGHT-ARM ROPE PULL DOWNS** *5 sets, 60 seconds' rest after each set*	25x
4	**GOOD MORNING BARBELL**	8x
5	**HYPEREXTENSION** (with optional 5- or 10-kilo weight)	12x
6	**SEATED ROW** *5 sets, 60 seconds' rest after each set*	25x
7	15 min. on treadmill, speed 80/110	

DAY 5 *Shoulders*

1	**SHOULDER PRESS**	8x
2	**FRONT RAISES**	12x
3	**SIDE LATERAL RAISES** *5 sets, 60 seconds' rest after each set*	25x
4	**STANDING INTERNAL ROTATION** each arm	8x
5	**PUSH UPS WIDE**	12x
6	**UPRIGHT ROW** *5 sets, 60 seconds' rest after each set*	25x
7	25 min. walking on treadmill with incline setting 13, speed 6)	

Phase 3 WEEK 9–12
5 DAYS' TRAINING

Supersets: 6 repetitions, as demanding as possible!

DAY 2 *Triceps & glutes*

#	Exercise	Reps
1	**DIPS** feet on bench and 5-kilo weight (minimum) on your legs	6x
2	**TRICEPS TRIANGLE PUSH DOWN** *5 sets, 60 seconds' rest after each set*	6x
3	**OVERHEAD ROPE PUSH**	6x
4	**DUMBBELL KICKBACK** *5 sets, 60 seconds' rest after each set*	6x
5	**INCLINE CHEST PRESS**	6x
6	**INCLINE FLYS** *5 sets, 60 seconds' rest after each set*	6x
7	**FLAT MACHINE PRESS**	6x
8	**PUSH UPS** *5 sets, 60 seconds' rest after each set*	6x

DAY 1 *Biceps & legs*

#	Exercise	Reps
1	**STANDING BARBELL BICEPS CURL**	6x
2	**HAMMER CURL** *5 sets, 60 seconds' rest after each set*	6x
3	**LYING BICEPS CURL**	6x
4	**SEATED DUMBBELL BICEPS CURL** *5 sets, 60 seconds' rest after each set*	6x
5	**HIP THRUSTER**	6x
6	**KETTLEBELL SUMO SQUAT** *5 sets, 60 seconds' rest after each set*	6x
7	**SMITH MACHINE DONKEY KICKS** each leg	6x
8	**LEG PRESS SMITH MACHINE** *5 sets, 60 seconds' rest after each set*	6x

DAY 3 *Legs*

#	Exercise	Reps
1	**FRONT SQUAT**	6x
2	**FROG JUMPS** each leg *5 sets, 60 seconds' rest after each set*	6x
3	**HAMSTRING CURLS**	6x
4	**LEG EXTENSION** *5 sets, 60 seconds' rest after each set*	6x
5	**SINGLE LEG SQUAT** foot on bench	6x
6	**STIFF-LEG DEADLIFT** *5 sets, 60 seconds' rest after each set*	6x
7	**WALKING LUNGES** each leg	6x
8	**STEP-UP BLOCK** each leg *5 sets, 60 seconds' rest after each set*	6x

DAY 4 *Back*

1 PULL UPS (6x)

2 WIDE GRIP LAT PULL DOWN (6x)
5 sets, 60 seconds' rest after each set

3 HYPEREXTENSION (6x)

4 ONE-ARM DUMBBELL ROW (6x)
each arm
5 sets, 60 seconds' rest after each set

5 SEATED ROW (6x)

6 BARBBELL PULL OVER (6x)
5 sets, 60 seconds' rest after each set

7 20 min. on treadmill, speed 80/110

DAY 5 *Shoulders & triceps*

1 SHOULDER PRESS (6x)

2 UPRIGHT ROW (6x)
5 sets, 60 seconds' rest after each set

3 SIDE RAISES (6x)

4 FRONT RAISES (6x)
5 sets, 60 seconds' rest after each set

5 REAR CABLE DELT FLYES (6x)

6 PUSH UPS (6x)
5 sets, 60 seconds' rest after each set

7 25 min. on treadmill with incline setting 13, speed 6

WESLEY VAN STAVEREN

The sports diet (page 106–111) and the training schedules for the gym (page 150–163) have been devised by Wesley van Staveren, a very experienced trainer, mentor and nutrition expert. He assists Fajah Lourens with the development of training programmes and information about nutrition and nutritional supplements.

Wesley is active in classic bodybuilding and is a 3-time European champion, 1-time world champion and winner of several international Grand Prix events. He coaches a number of athletes in a variety of disciplines and leagues. Having developed his expertise over many years he is well-qualified to provide advice on nutrition, nutritional supplements and training.

IV

RECIPES

All calories and nutritional breakdowns are per single serving.

Breakfast

Salads

Snacks

Soup

Dinner

Smoothies

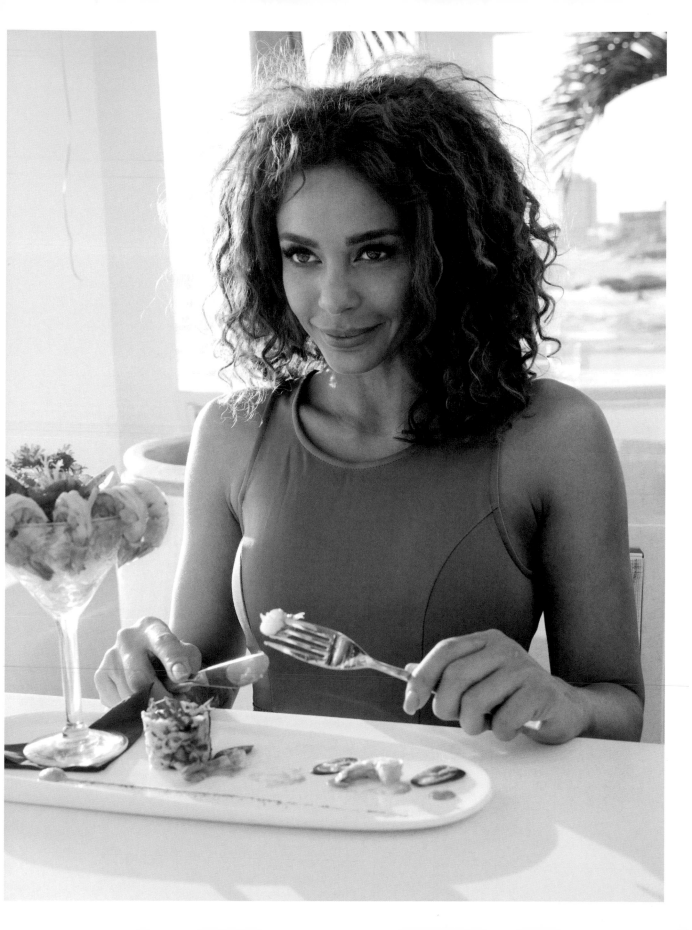

Breakfast
OVERNIGHT OATS

317 kcal

FAT 7.53 g

CARBS 47.7 g

PROTEIN 10.88 g

INGREDIENTS
Serves one

40 g rolled oats

100 ml almond milk

juice of ½ lemon

fresh fruit of your choice

PREPARATION

1 Put the oats in a bowl.

2 Add milk and stir.

3 Cover and put in the fridge overnight to soak.

4 Add the lemon juice and stir through.

5 Serve with blueberries or other fresh fruit.

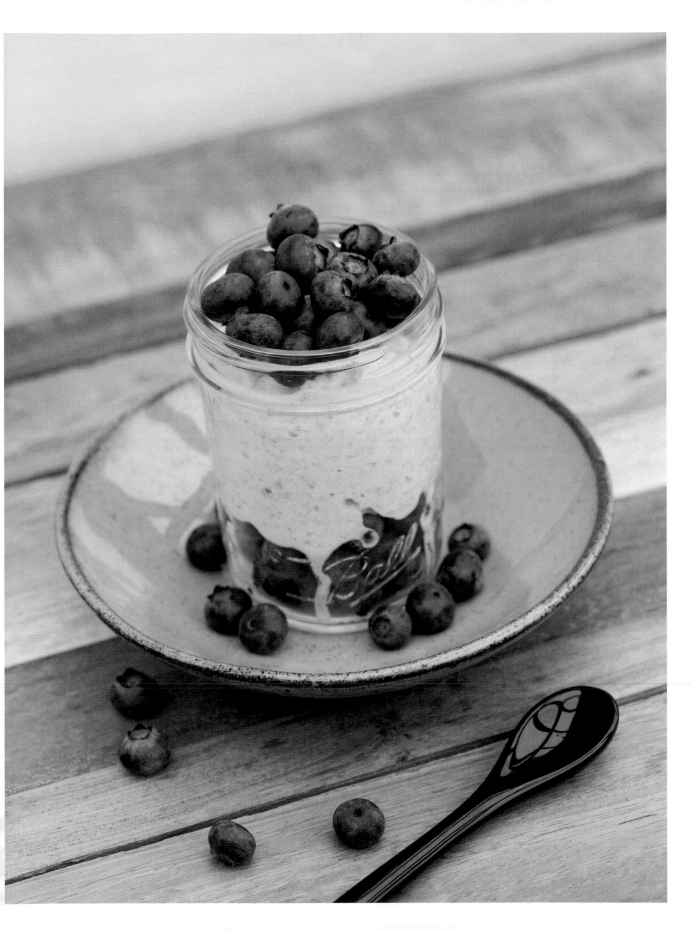

Breakfast
PROTEIN PANCAKES

431 kcal

FAT 15.55 g

CARBS 34.95 g

PROTEIN 38.54 g

INGREDIENTS
Serves one

3 eggs

30 g rolled oats

½ banana

1 scoop vanilla protein

1 teaspoon coconut oil

PREPARATION

1 Separate the yolks from two of the eggs.

2 Put the two egg whites plus one whole egg in a bowl and mix.

3 Add the rolled oats, banana and the protein.

4 Mix thoroughly and fry in coconut oil, like a pancake.

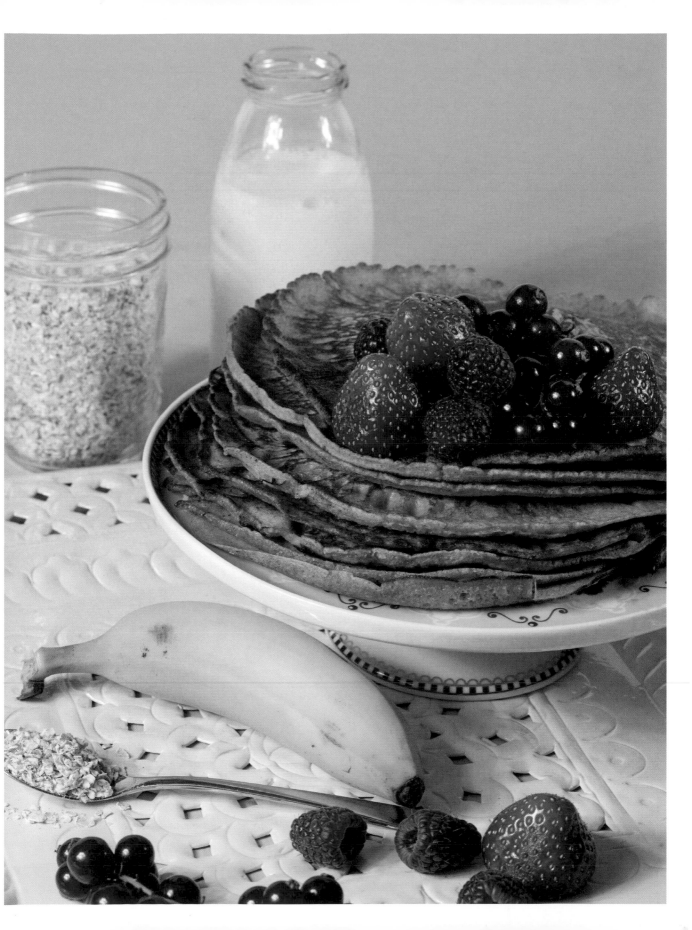

Salad
TUNA SALAD

129 kcal

FAT 4.10 g

CARBS 4.64 g

PROTEIN 15.92 g

INGREDIENTS
Serves two

1 handful of cherry tomatoes

1 handful of radishes

½ cucumber

150 g salad leaves

100 g cooked French beans

10–15 black olives

1 tin of tuna

pepper and salt

PREPARATION

1 Slice the tomatoes, radishes and cucumber, and combine with salad leaves.

2 Garnish with the beans and olives.

3 Add the tinned tuna and season with pepper and salt.

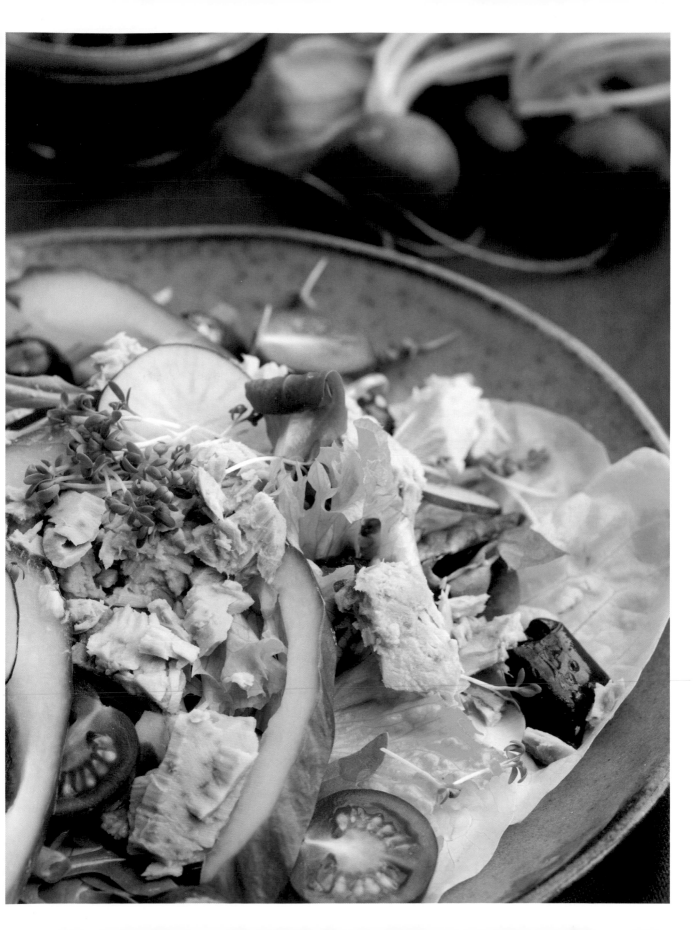

Salad

CHICKEN SALAD

403 kcal

FAT 21.09 g

CARBS 6.65 g

PROTEIN 43.21 g

INGREDIENTS
Serves two

200 g lambs lettuce

1 avocado

2 cherry tomatoes

250 g chicken breast

100 g mushrooms

pepper and salt

PREPARATION

1 Arrange the lettuce on two plates.

2 Slice the avocado and tomato, and scatter over the lettuce.

3 Cube the chicken, and fry till golden and cooked through.

4 Fry the mushrooms.

5 Place the fried chicken and mushrooms on top of the salad.

6 Add salt and pepper to taste.

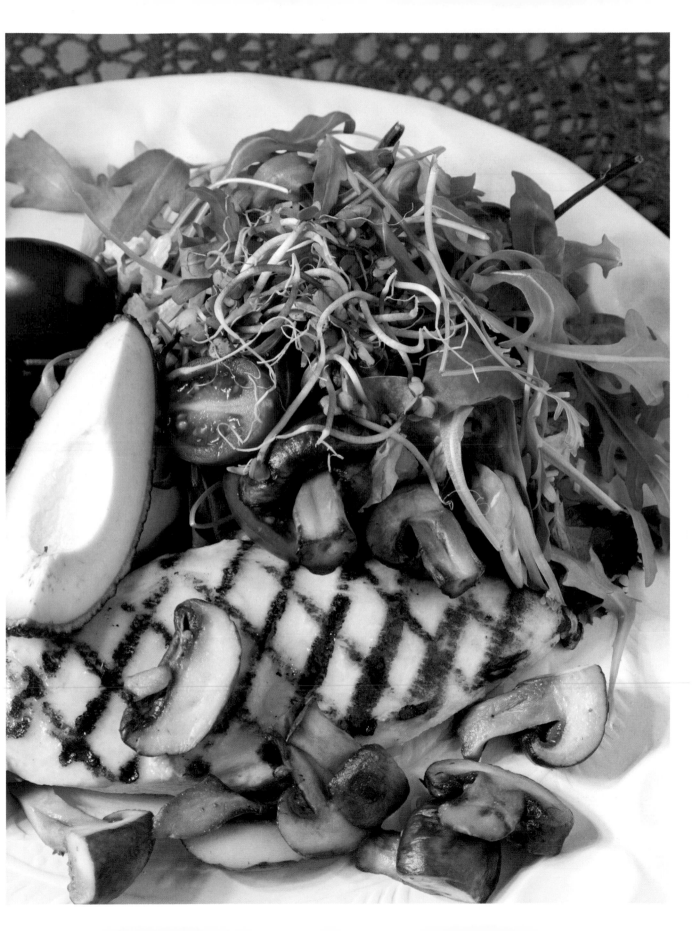

Salad
VEGAN SALAD

305 kcal

FAT 17.16 g

CARBS 17.96 g

PROTEIN 15.23 g

INGREDIENTS
Serves two

200 g mixed salad leaves

2 boiled eggs, sliced in half

100 g sweetcorn

100 g chickpeas (tinned)

1 pepper, chopped

1 handful of walnuts

1 tablespoon olive oil

PREPARATION

1 Arrange the salad leaves on two plates.

2 Scatter all remaining ingredients over the top.

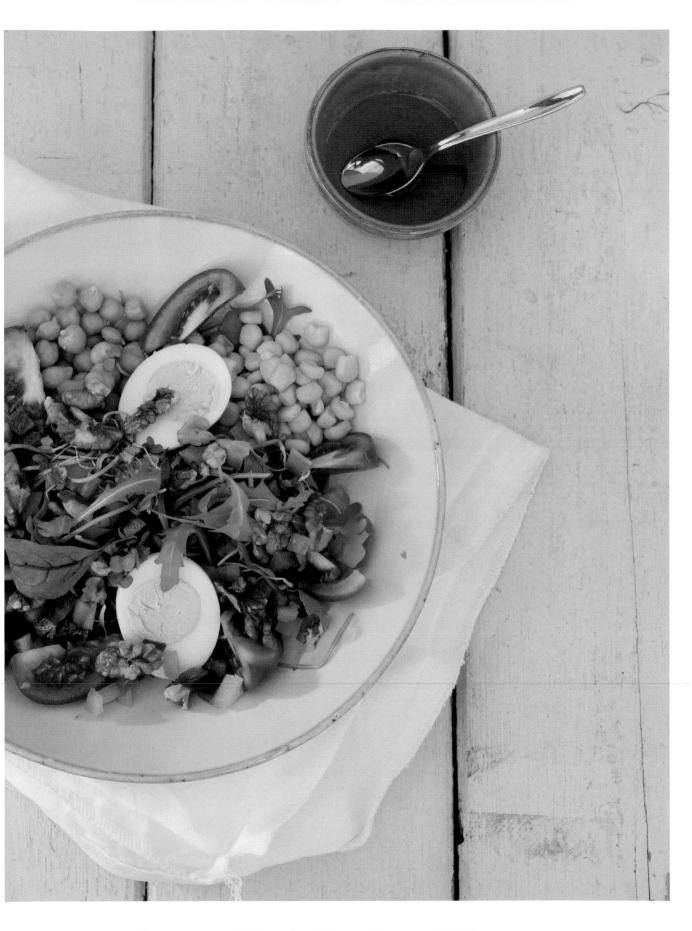

Snack

CHOCO– VANILLA PROTEIN BALLS

TIP
Any leftover protein balls can be frozen for later use.

FOR AFTER THE 12-WEEK PLAN

INGREDIENTS
Makes around 19 balls

200 g pitted dates

50 g raisins

50 g (peeled) pistachios

50 g pumpkin seeds

150 g almonds

50 g (melted) coconut oil

1 tablespoon raw cocoa powder

1 teaspoon vanilla powder

1 scoop vanilla-flavoured protein powder

pinch of salt

138 kcal (per ball)

FAT 11.21 g

CARBS 11.99 g

PROTEIN 5.06 g

PREPARATION

1 Blend all the ingredients in a food processor until they form a dough-like consistency.

2 Roll the mixture into little 2–3cm balls. Eat straight away or put in the fridge to set for 1–2 hours.

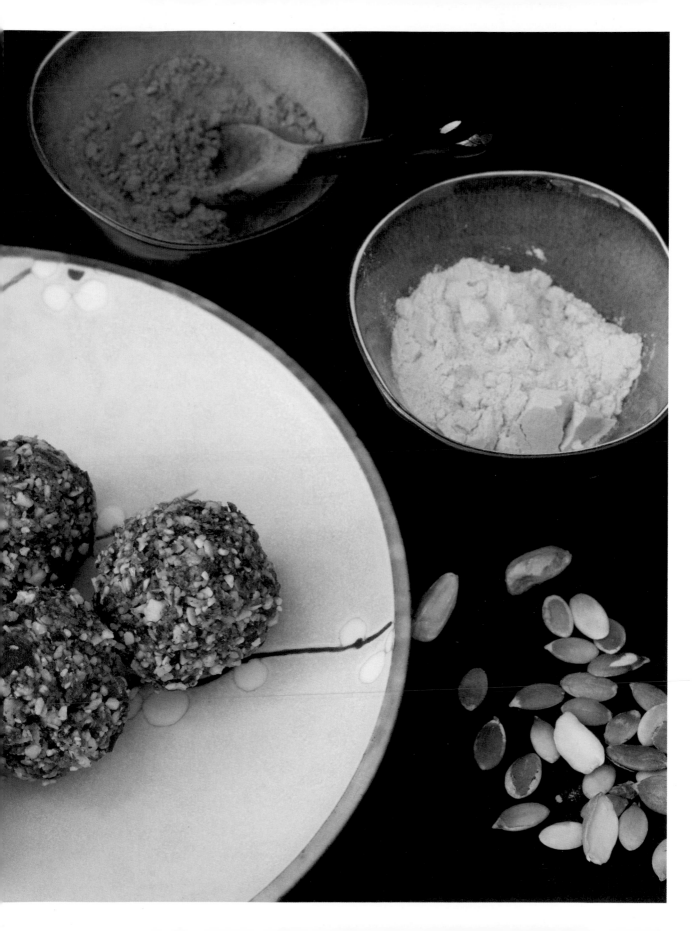

Soup

PUMPKIN & SWEET POTATO SOUP

304 kcal (per person as main dish)

FAT 11.4 g

CARBS 42.95 g

PROTEIN 4.03 g

INGREDIENTS
Serves four

1 small pumpkin

1 red onion, sliced

1 garlic clove, diced

1 tablespoon coconut oil

2 sweet potatoes, chopped

½ red chilli pepper, sliced

2 coriander sprigs

1 litre vegetable stock

salt

PREPARATION

1 Halve the pumpkin, remove seeds and cut into small pieces.

2 In a stock pot, gently fry the onion and garlic in coconut oil.

3 Add the pieces of pumpkin, sweet potato, chilli and coriander sprigs, and gently fry for another 5 minutes.

4 Add the vegetable stock and slowly bring the mixture to the boil, then simmer for about 25 minutes or until the sweet potatoes are very soft.

5 Remove the coriander.

6 Blend the soup using either a hand blender or food processor.

7 Add salt to taste.

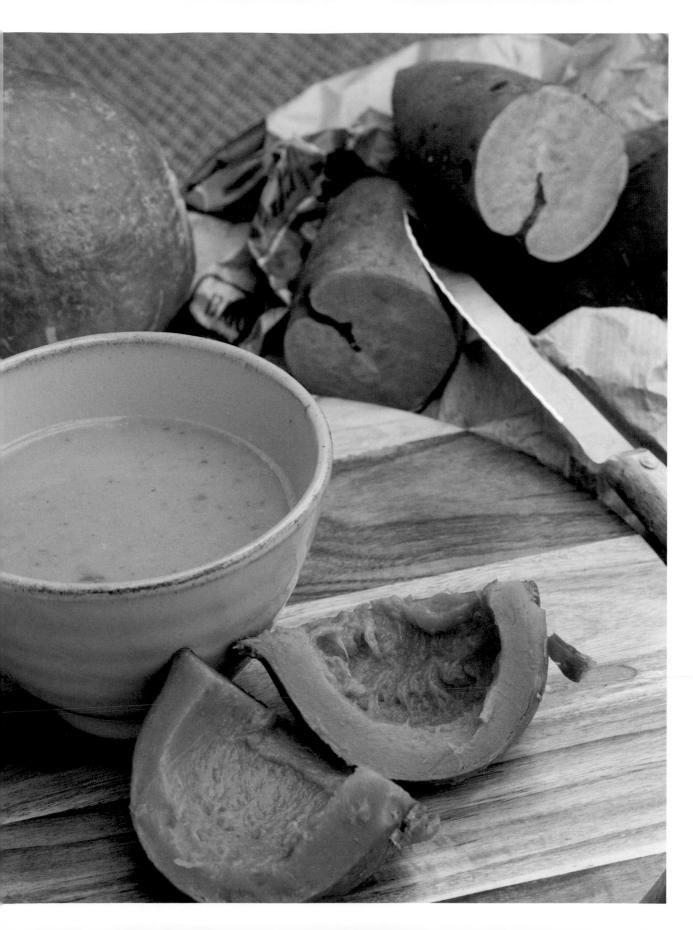

Soup
GREEN SOUP

128 kcal

FAT 6.12 g

CARBS 8.04 g

PROTEIN 7.82 g

INGREDIENTS
Serves four

2 broccoli heads

2 courgettes

1 litre stock

pepper and salt

200 g mushrooms, sliced)

1 tablespoon coconut oil

PREPARATION

1 Cut the broccoli into smaller rosettes and slice the courgette. Boil briefly and save some of the cooking liquid.

2 Put the boiled vegetables and some of the liquid into a food processor, blending until smooth.

3 Return mixture to the stock pot and add the stock.

4 Leave on a low simmer for a while; add pepper and salt to taste. The thickness of the soup will depend on how much stock you add.

5 Fry the mushrooms in coconut oil.

6 Ladle the soup into bowls and garnish with the fried mushrooms.

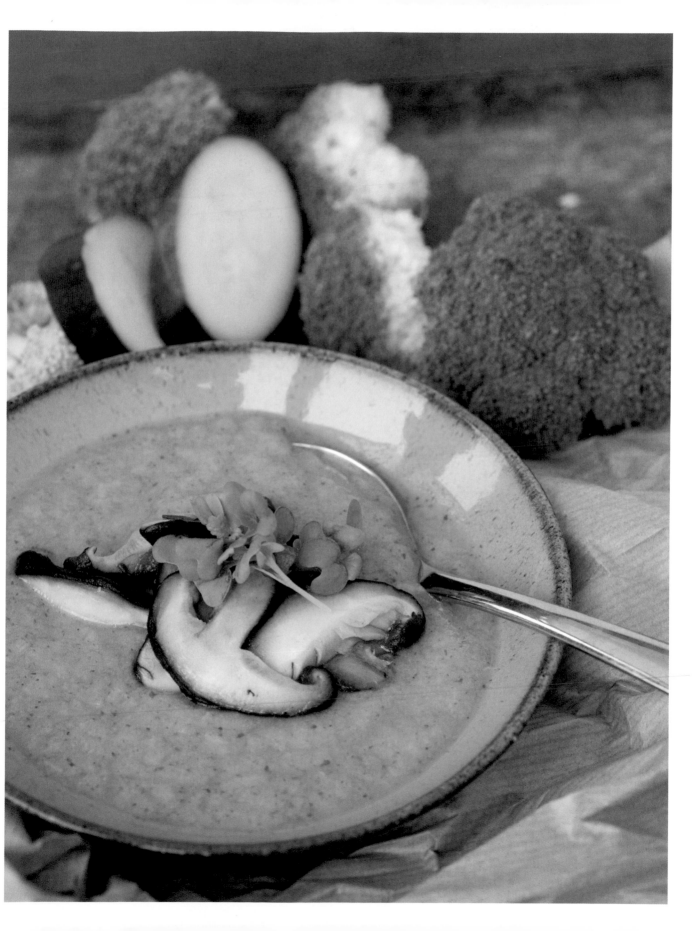

Dinner
VEGETARIAN LASAGNE

FOR AFTER THE
12-WEEK PLAN

388 kcal

FAT 23.07 g

CARBS 15.64 g

PROTEIN 27.85 g

INGREDIENTS
Serves two

1 courgette, sliced

1 aubergine, sliced

1 onion, sliced

1 red pepper, sliced

olive oil (for greasing)

2 tomatoes, sliced

2 mozzarella balls, sliced

Italian herbs

tomato sauce

pepper and salt

PREPARATION

1 Grill the courgette, aubergine, onion and pepper in a grill pan. Grease an oven dish with olive oil.

2 Alternate layers of grilled vegetables (coated in olive oil if preferred), tomato, mozzarella, Italian herbs, pepper and salt, using a little of the tomato sauce to cover each layer.

3 Top the final layer with more mozzarella slices according to preference.

4 Cook for 35–40 minutes in an oven preheated to 175ºC.

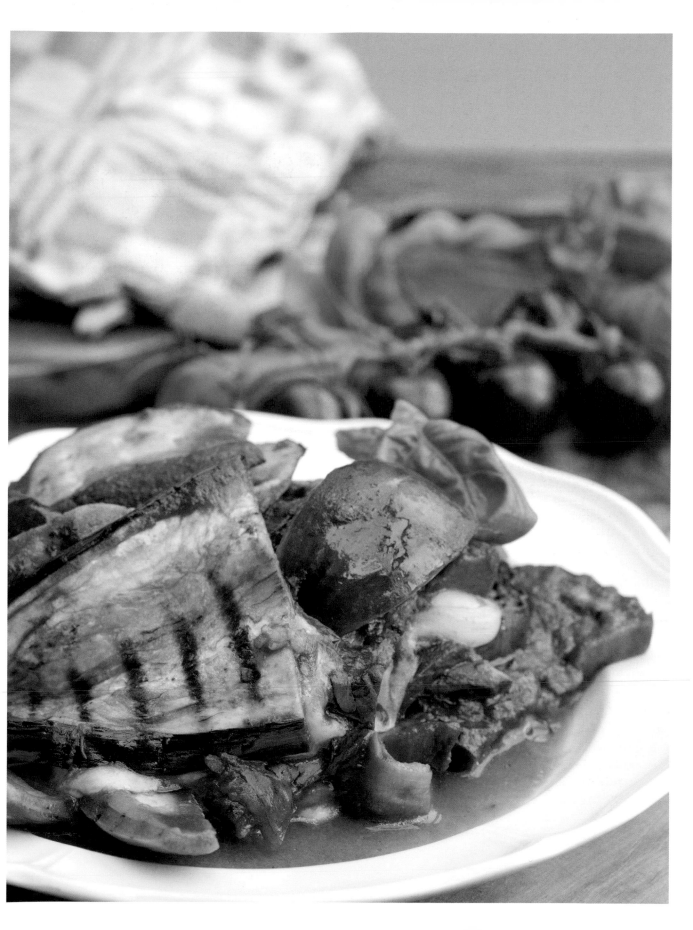

Bases

BOLOGNESE SAUCE

386 kcal (these values apply to the sauce only, i.e. without the pasta)

FAT 24 g

CARBS 12.40 g

PROTEIN 27.85 g

TIP
This will serve one person for the whole of Phase 1; it can be frozen in separate portions.

INGREDIENTS
Serves four

20 g butter

20 g olive oil

2 onions, chopped

2 garlic cloves, chopped

500 g lean ground beef

1 kg ripe tomatoes

1 handful of basil

50 g tomato purée

pepper and salt

extra vegetables (optional)

PREPARATION

1 Melt the butter and olive oil in a large pan. Add the onion and garlic, and gently fry until soft.

2 Add the beef, frying until browned.

3 Add the tomatoes and basil, turn up the heat a little and let it simmer. Keep stirring and, as the tomatoes soften, press them with a wooden spoon to break them down.

4 Stir the tomato purée through the mixture then leave to simmer. Add salt and pepper to taste.

5 You can add any other stir-fried vegetables of your choice to the base sauce, for example carrots, courgettes, peppers etc.

6 Serve with your favourite pasta.

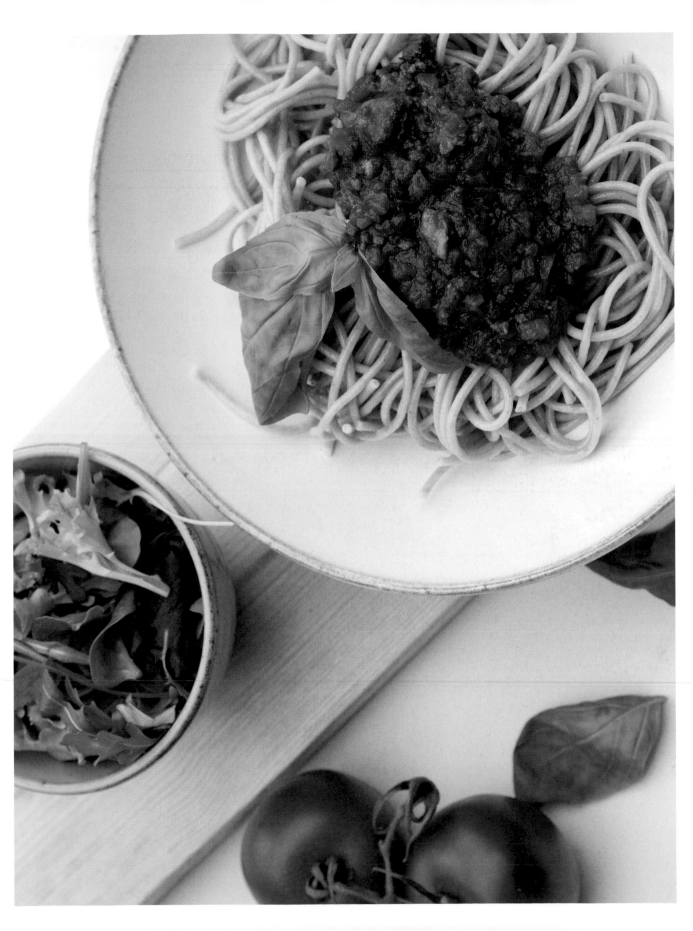

Dinner

OVEN–BAKED CHICKEN

FAJAH'S MOTHER–IN–LAW'S RECIPE

387 kcal (based on 150 g chicken breast per person)

FAT 15.04 g

CARBS 2.23 g

PROTEIN 60.48 g

INGREDIENTS
Serves four

4 chicken breast fillets

a few slices of Serrano ham or bacon (per person)

½ onion, sliced

2 garlic cloves, thinly sliced

Genovese pesto

pine nuts

pepper and salt

PREPARATION

1 Season the fillets with salt (optional) and pepper.

2 Lay out the slices of ham or bacon, slightly overlapping.

3 Cover with the onion and garlic.

4 Brush one side of the fillets with pesto and lay on top of the ham/bacon (pesto-side down).

5 Brush the other side of the chicken breasts with pesto and cover them lengthwise with 2 slices of ham/bacon, again slightly overlapping.

6 Lay the fillets 'right' side up in an oven dish. Sprinkle with pine nuts and cover the dish with foil. Bake in a preheated oven at 180°C for 25 minutes.

7 Remove the foil and bake for another 10 minutes.

You can also use red pesto and red onion, for example, and sundried tomatoes or finely chopped leek. If you make small incisions in the fillets and insert the garlic slices, it will flavour the meat even better.

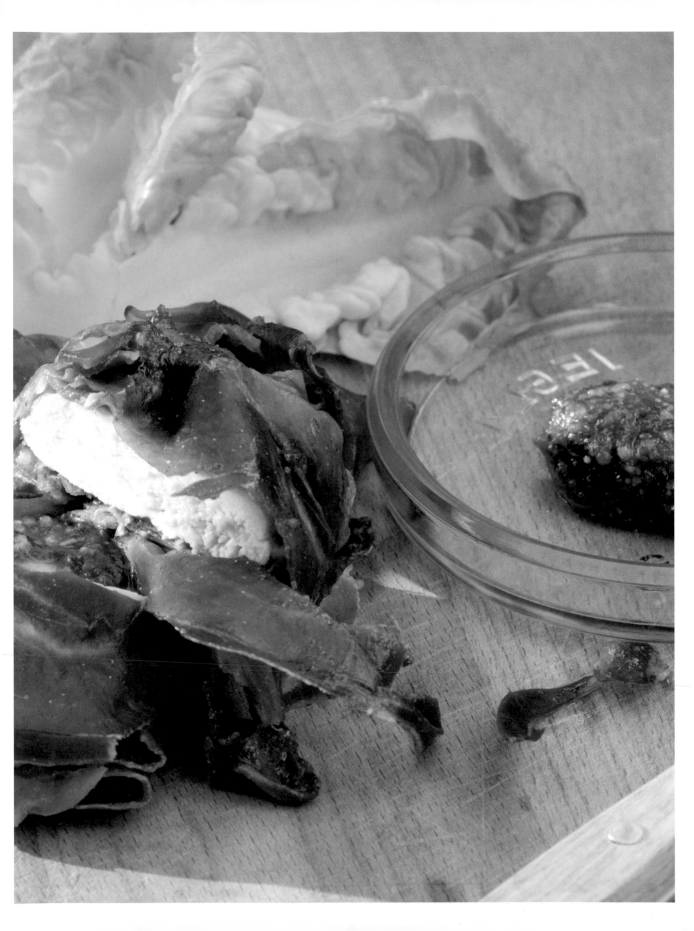

Dinner
HAMBURGER

252 kcal

FAT 14.71 g

CARBS 3.05 g

PROTEIN 26.30 g

INGREDIENTS
Serves four

500 g lean ground beef

1 garlic clove, finely sliced

1 onion, finely sliced

1 egg yolk

1 tablespoon ketjap (Indonesian sweet soy sauce)

1 teaspoon mustard

pepper and salt

tomato (optional, for topping)

extra onion (optional, for topping)

gherkin (optional, for topping)

PREPARATION

1 Combine the ground beef with all the other ingredients in a bowl and mix thoroughly.

2 Shape into four balls (125 g each) and flatten into hamburgers.

3 Fry the burgers for 3–4 minutes on both sides.

4 Put the burger on top of a bun or perhaps try lettuce leaves as an alternative base.

5 Top with tomato, onion, gherkin etc.

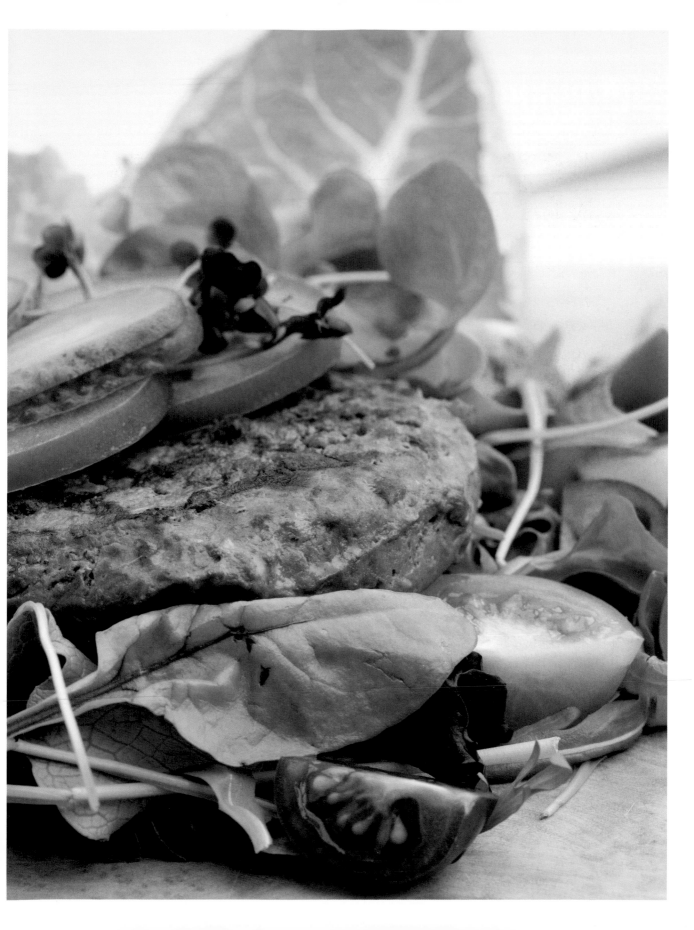

Dinner

COURGETTE SPAGHETTI & CREAM CHEESE

293 kcal

FAT 14.48 g

CARBS 13.57 g

PROTEIN 25.64 g

INGREDIENTS
Serves two

1 courgette

1 red onion, diced

1 garlic clove, diced

200 g smoked chicken, chopped

1 spring onion, chopped

100 g of light cream cheese

pepper and salt

PREPARATION

1 Use a spiralizer to turn the courgette into spaghetti noodles or slice it thinly.

2 Gently fry the red onion and garlic.

3 Add the smoked chicken and spring onion then fry for a few more minutes.

4 Add the cream cheese and stir through, adding salt and pepper to taste.

5 In another pan quickly fry the courgette spaghetti.

6 Serve the courgette spaghetti with the cream cheese sauce.

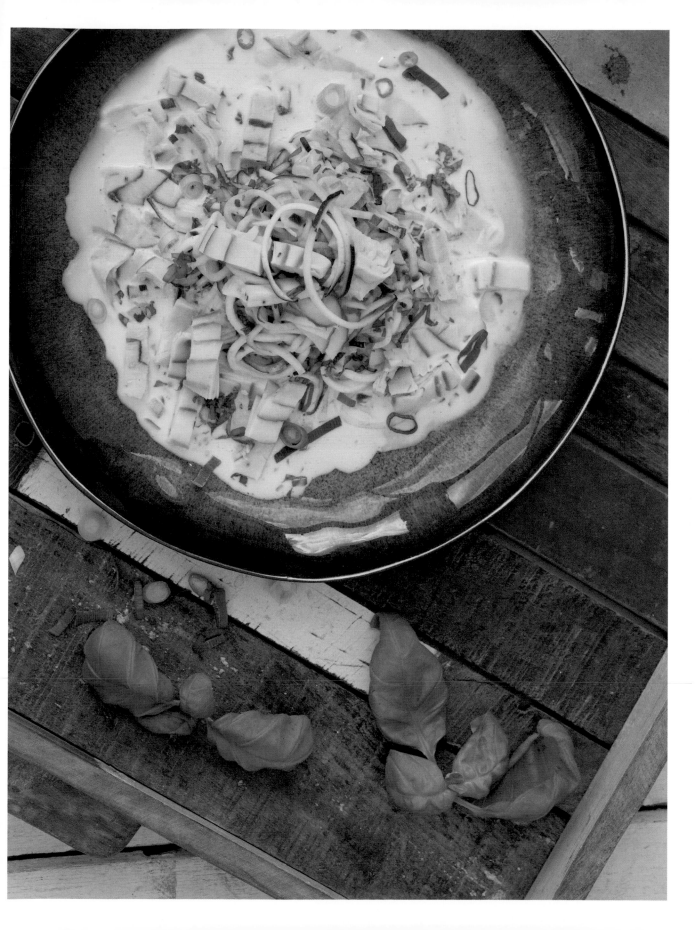

Dinner

SPICY PENNE & SMOKED TROUT

520 kcal

FAT 31.7 g

CARBS 40.19 g

PROTEIN 30.92 g

INGREDIENTS
Serves two

100 g wholegrain penne pasta

1 leek, sliced

2 garlic cloves, chopped

½ red chilli pepper, chopped

1 tomato, chopped

100 ml crème fraiche

150 g smoked trout

pumpkin seeds

PREPARATION

1 Cook the penne as per the instructions on the pack.

2 Fry the leek with the garlic, chilli and tomato.

3 Stir in the crème fraiche and heat through.

4 Pour the sauce over the penne and garnish with the smoked trout.

5 Sprinkle pumpkin seeds on top.

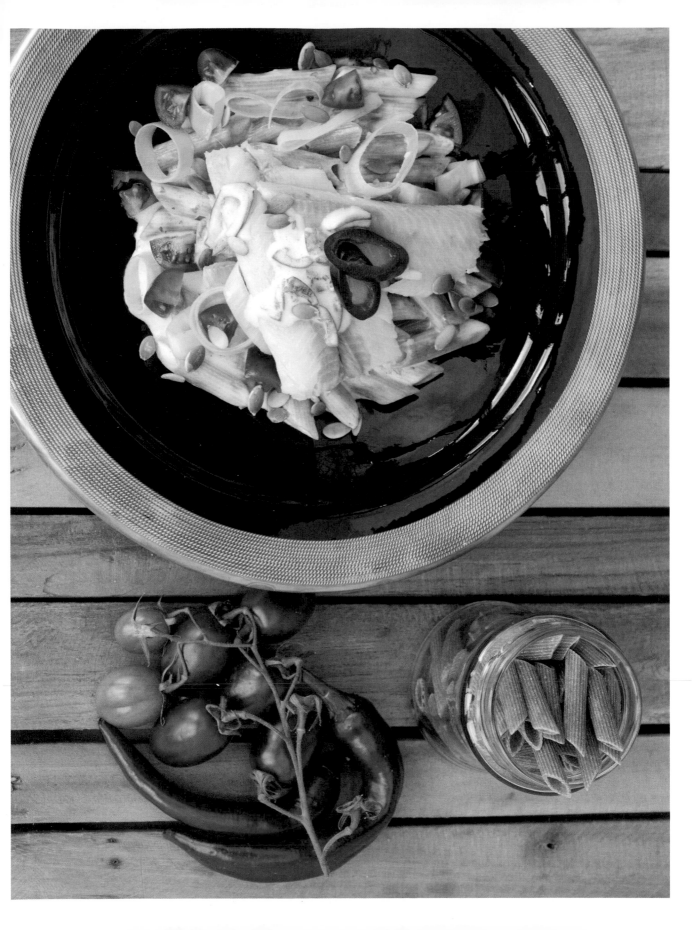

Smoothie
FOR AFTER THE 12-WEEK PLAN

WATER–MELON CUCUMBER SPINACH

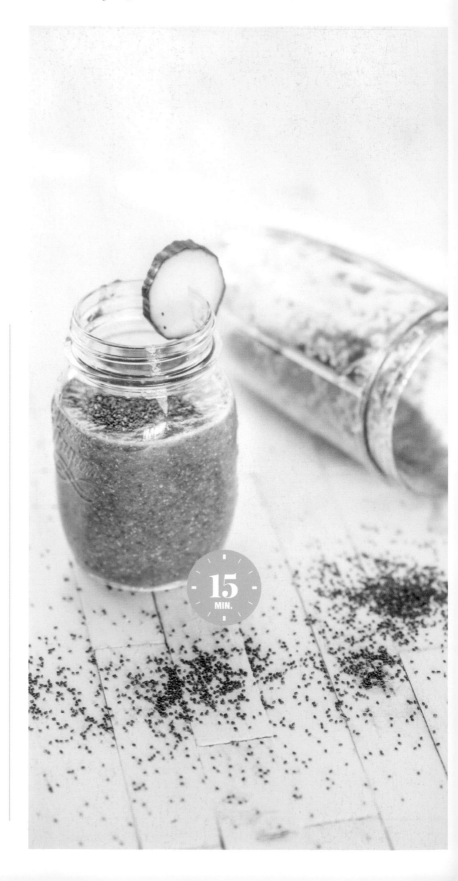

INGREDIENTS
Makes 3–4 glasses

150 g watermelon pieces

150 g diced cucumber

675 g fresh spinach

2 tablespoons baobab powder*

1 tablespoon chia seeds

1 tablespoon fresh basil leaves

120 ml water

* available online

PREPARATION

Combine all ingredients and blend for 1–2 minutes until smooth.

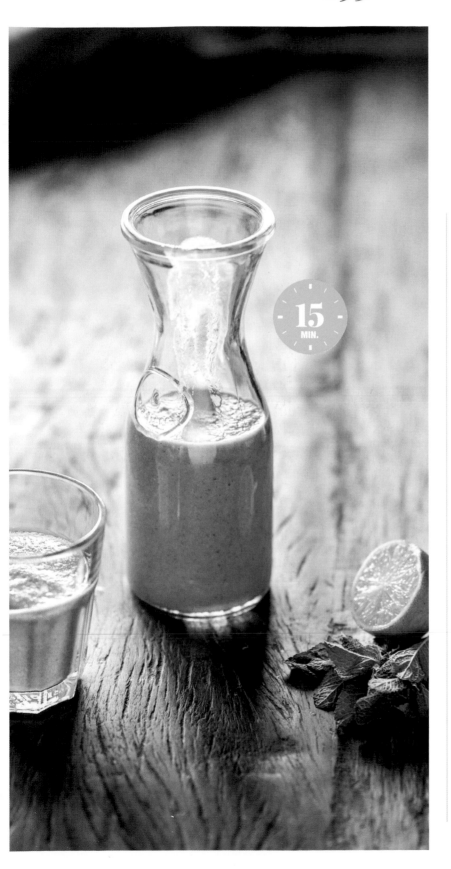

Smoothie
FOR AFTER THE 12-WEEK PLAN

SWEET ANTI- OXIDANT

INGREDIENTS
Makes 3–4 glasses

1 banana, sliced

450 g cantaloupe melon pieces

½ diced cucumber

1 tablespoon Vitamineral Green (superfood powder)*

1 tablespoon baobab powder*

1 tablespoon camu powder*

1 teaspoon vanilla essence

juice of ½ lime

3 sprigs fresh mint

* available online

PREPARATION

Combine all ingredients and blend for 1–2 minutes until smooth

Smoothie
FOR AFTER THE 12-WEEK PLAN

ALOE–CUCUMBER

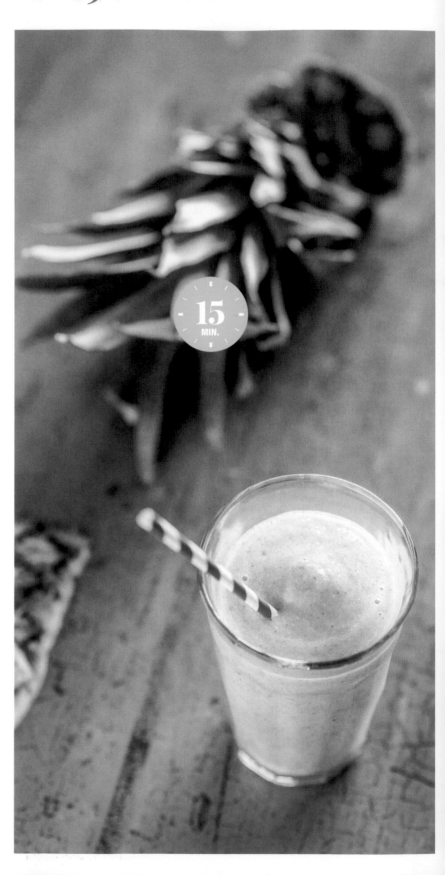

INGREDIENTS
Makes three glasses

450 g pineapple pieces

450 g diced cucumber

25 g parsley

2 tablespoons baobab powder*

2 tablespoons chia seeds

120 ml aloe vera juice*

optional: add some fennel slices for a fuller flavour

* available online

PREPARATION

Combine all the ingredients and blend for 1–2 minutes until smooth.

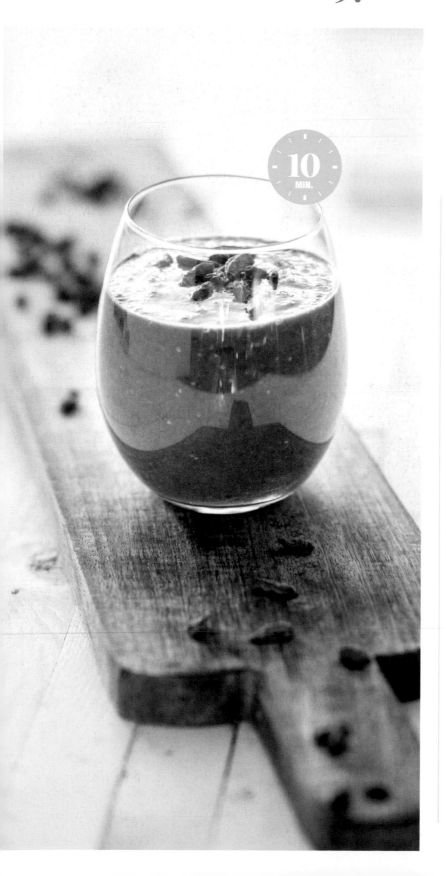

Smoothie
FOR AFTER THE 12-WEEK PLAN

BODY & MIND

INGREDIENTS
Makes two glasses

525 g orange segments

2 tablespoons aloe vera gel (bottled)*

2 tablespoons goji berries (rehydrated)

1 tablespoon raw cocoa powder

1 teaspoon camu powder*

1 teaspoon chaga powder*

1 teaspoon fresh ginger

5 dates, cut into small pieces

topping: raw cocoa nibs

* available online

PREPARATION

Combine all the ingredients and blend for 1–2 minutes until smooth. Sprinkle the cocoa nibs on top.

Smoothie
FOR AFTER THE 12-WEEK PLAN
SLIM BODY

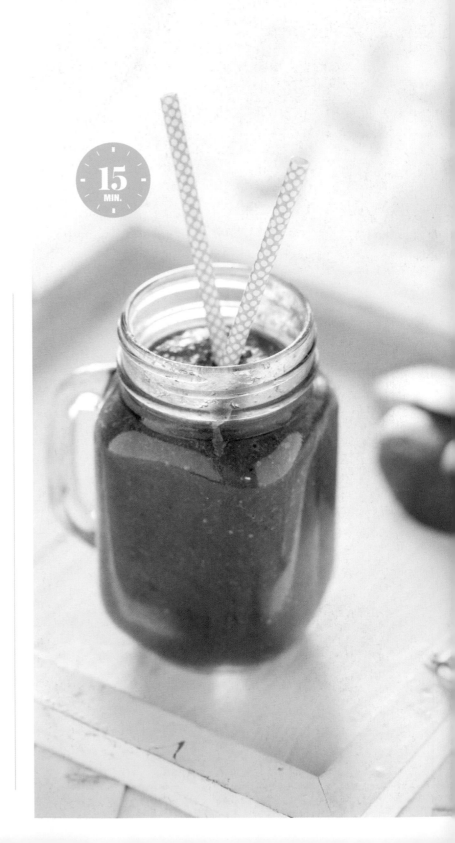

INGREDIENTS
Makes two glasses

1 mango, cut into pieces

⅓ watermelon, cut into pieces

20 fresh mint leaves

3 tablespoons goji berries, rehydrated

2 tablespoons baobab powder*

1 tablespoon acai powder*

240 ml red grape juice

* available online

PREPARATION

Combine all the ingredients and blend for 1–2 minutes until smooth.

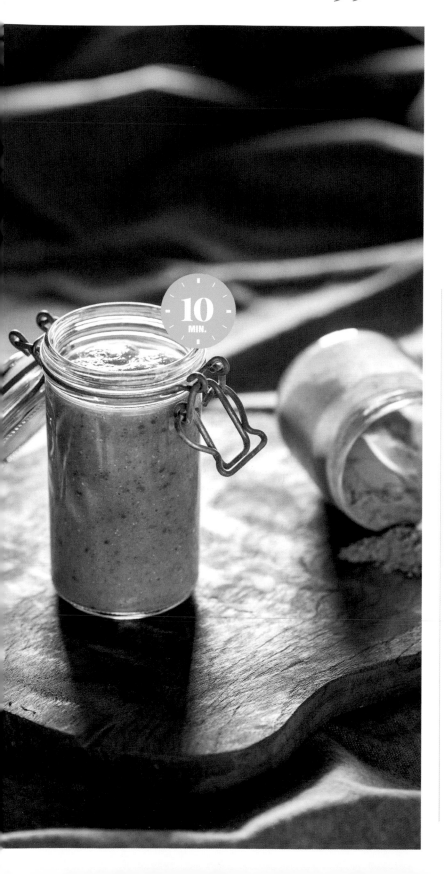

10 MIN.

Smoothie
Smoothie
FOR AFTER THE
12-WEEK PLAN

DRAGON FRUIT 'WEIGH LESS'

INGREDIENTS
Makes two glasses

150 g dragon fruit (pitaya)
or apple pieces

1 banana, sliced

150 g mango pieces

2 tablespoons aloe vera gel
(bottled)*

1 tablespoon barley grass
powder*

150 g frozen almond milk
cubes

* available online

PREPARATION

Cut the dragon fruit in half
and scoop out the flesh.
Combine with the other
ingredients and blend for
1–2 minutes until smooth.

Smoothie
FOR AFTER THE 12-WEEK PLAN

ICY MACA

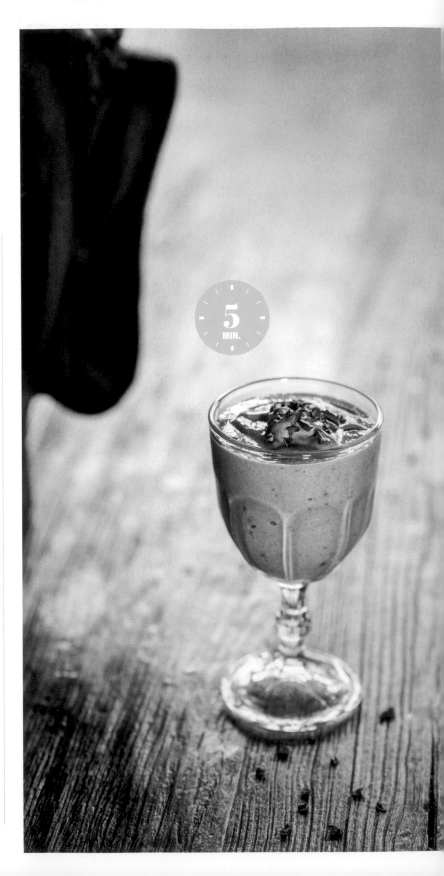

INGREDIENTS
Makes two glasses

1 banana, sliced

2 tablespoons raw cocoa powder

3 tablespoons maca powder

2 tablespoons hemp seeds (peeled)

1 teaspoon cinnamon

12 drops Stevia or 1 tablespoon maple syrup

300 g frozen almond milk cubes

PREPARATION

Combine all ingredients and blend for 1–2 minutes until smooth.

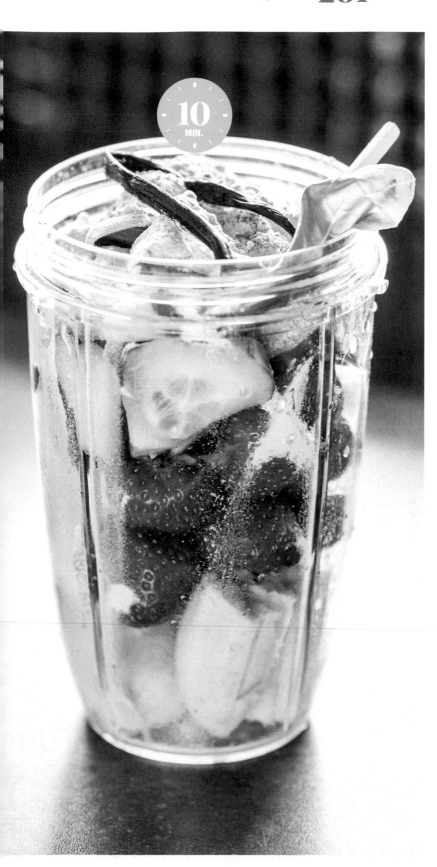

Smoothie
FOR AFTER THE 12-WEEK PLAN

MUSCLES & BONES

INGREDIENTS
Makes two glasses

2 bananas, sliced

750 g strawberries

½ cucumber, diced

55 g lettuce leaves

1 handful of dill sprigs

1 handful of basil leaves

1 tablespoon maca powder

1 tablespoon baobab powder

½ teaspoon cinnamon powder

½ vanilla pod (scrape out the inside)

PREPARATION

Combine all ingredients and blend for 1–2 minutes until smooth.

10 MIN.

Smoothie
FOR AFTER THE 12-WEEK PLAN

NO MORE BRAINFOG

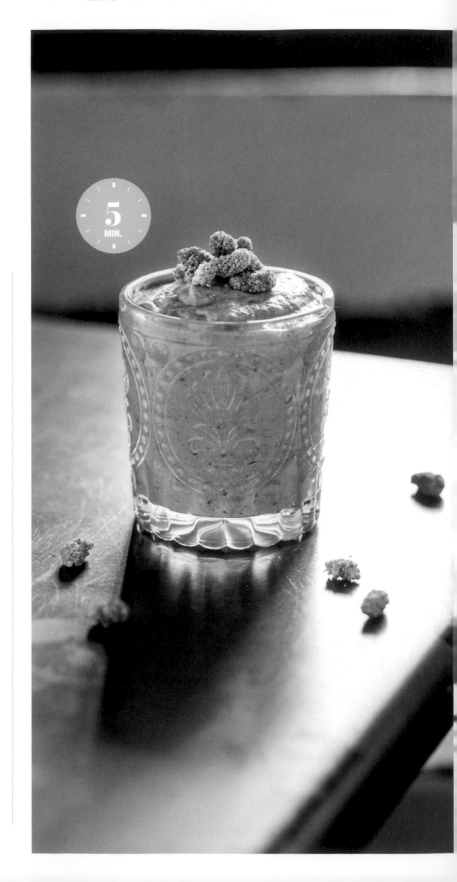

5 MIN.

INGREDIENTS
Makes two glasses

100 g redcurrants

150 g red gooseberries

1 tablespoon hemp seeds, peeled

2 tablespoons lucuma powder*

3 tablespoons strawberry powder

240 ml rice or coconut milk

topping: black or white mulberries

* available online

PREPARATION

Combine all ingredients and blend for 1–2 minutes until smooth. Sprinkle the mulberries on top.

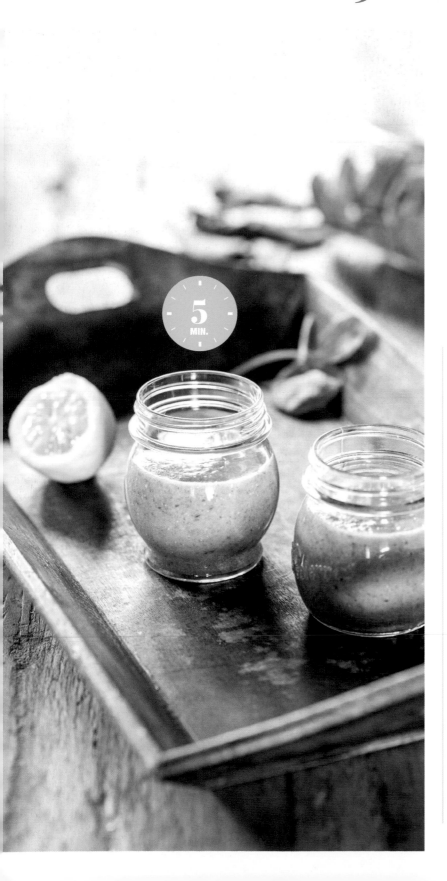

Smoothie
FOR AFTER THE
12-WEEK PLAN

SECOND TRIMESTER SMOOTHIE
(DURING PREGNANCY)

INGREDIENTS
Makes two glasses

½ banana, sliced

juice of 1 lemon

150 g frozen peach pieces

150 ml organic pineapple juice

150 g fresh spinach

1 tablespoon chia seeds

6 medjool dates, cut into small pieces

PREPARATION

Combine all ingredients and blend for 1–2 minutes until smooth.

Shopping list

These are the items you need per person, per week, during each phase. It is assumed that you will have the following 'staple' items already: pepper, salt, olive oil, coconut oil, ketjap (a sweet Indonesian soy sauce), mustard, Genovese pesto, honey, cinnamon powder, peanut butter, butter, red onions, fresh garlic, and casein protein (www.MKBMshop. com, Enter code: MKBMproteine for a 10% discount), vitamin D, a multivitamin and fish oil capsules. Any leftovers can be frozen for later use (during the same phase).

PHASE 1

Almond milk (100 ml)
Apples (6)
Asparagus bunch
Avocadoes (3)
Bananas
Beef tartare (80 g)
Breadsticks (1)
Broccoli (200 g)
Capers (optional)
Cherry tomatoes
Chicken breast (225 g)
Chickpeas (tinned, 50 g)
Cocoa powder (optional)
Cooked chicken breast
   (8 slices)
Cottage cheese (190 g)
Courgette (1)
Cream cheese (light,
   about 60 g)
Crème fraiche (50 ml)
Cucumber (3)
Eggs (17)
Fresh fruit (any)
Greek yogurt 0% fat
   (200 ml)
Green beans (50 g)
Houmous (10 g)
Lean ground beef
   (100 g)

Leek (½)
Lemons (1)
Lettuce/salad leaves
   (275 g)
Light crackers (6)
Low-fat flavoured Quark
   (200 g)
Low-fat Quark (350 g)
Wholegrain roll (1)
Mushrooms (50 g)
Oat flakes (40 g)
Orange (1)
Pepper (½)
Porridge/rolled oats
   (60 g)
Radishes (½ handful)
Red chilli pepper (¼)
Rice (240 g)
Runner beans (200 g)
Smoked chicken (100 g)
Smoked salmon (50 g)
Smoked trout (75 g)
Stir-fry vegetables
   (200 g)
Sweet potato (80 g)
Sweetcorn (50 g)
Tomatoes (3)
Tuna (½ tin)
Vanilla protein
   (2 scoops)

Walnuts (½ handful)
White fish (200 g)
Wholemeal bread
   (1 slice)
Wholemeal wraps
   (2 × 40 g)
Wholewheat penne
   (50 g)
1 × for this phase:
Black olives (5–8)
Fat-free broth
Pumpkin seeds (1 bag)

PHASE 2

Apples (5)
Aubergine (½)
Avocado (¾)
Bananas (1)
Basil (½ handful)
Breadsticks (4)
Broccoli (200 g)
Cherry tomatoes (about
   ½ handful)
Chicken breast (300 g)
Chicken breast
   (smoked, 50 g)
Chickpeas (tinned, 50 g)
Cooked chicken breast
   (22 slices)
Coriander (½ sprig)
Cottage cheese (30 g)
Courgette (1)
Cucumber (1¼)
Eggs (12)
Extra vegetables
   (optional)
Gherkin (optional)
Green beans (250 g)
Houmous (10 g)
Kiwi fruit (2)

Lean ground beef
   (425 g)
Lean (beef) meatballs
   (100 g)
Lemon (1)
Lettuce or salad leaves
   (175 g)
Light crackers (1)
Low-fat flavoured Quark
   (200 g)
Low-fat Quark (400 g)
Mozzarella (1 ball)
Mozzarella light (80 g)
Orange (1)
Pepper (1)
Pineapple (6 slices)
Porridge (60 g)
Pumpkin (¼)
Radishes (½ handful)
Rice (80 g)
Rice cakes (4)
Red chilli pepper (¼)
Smoked beef (80 g)
Serrano ham (a few
   slices)
Shrimp or chicken
   (100 g)
Spinach (200 g)
Sweet potato (100 g)
Sweetcorn (50 g)
Tomatoes (about 2 kg)
Tomato paste (25 g)
Tuna (½ tin)
Vegetable (any) (200 g)
Vegetables for soup
   (200 g)
Wholemeal bread (3
   slices)
Whey protein (20 g)
White fish (100 g)

Wholewheat pasta (80 g)

Wholemeal wraps (2 × 40 g)

1 × for this phase:

Black olives (1 jar)

Fat-free broth

Italian herbs

Pine nuts (1 bag)

Vanilla protein

Vegetable stock

Walnuts (1 bag)

PHASE 3

Apples (2)

Avocado (1)

Bananas (2)

Basil (½ handful)

Breadsticks (7)

Broccoli (½ head)

Carpaccio (100 g)

Cherry tomatoes (about 1 handful)

Chicken breast (450 g)

Cooked chicken breast (slices, 120 g)

Cottage cheese (150 g)

Courgette (½)

Cucumber (1¼)

Dates (2)

Eggs (16)

Extra vegetables (optional)

French fries (10)

Gherkin (optional)

Green beans (50 g)

Green vegetables (200 g)

Kiwi fruit (5)

Lean ground beef (200 g)

Lettuce/salad leaves (375 g)

Light crackers (4)

Low-fat Quark (600 g)

Low-fat yogurt (150 g)

Muesli (30 g)

Wholegrain roll (3)

Mushrooms (100 g)

Orange (2)

Porridge/rolled oats (100 g)

Radishes (½ handful)

Rice (160 g)

Rice cakes (2)

Roast beef (70 g)

Rocket leaves (200 g)

Runner beans (200 g)

Serrano ham (a few slices)

Shrimp or white fish (75 g)

Smoked beef (30 g)

Smoked fish (50 g or 2 herrings)

Spinach (200 g)

Stir-fry vegetables (200 g)

Sweet potato (80 g)

Tomato (about 600 g)

Tomato paste (25 g)

Tuna (½ tin)

Wholemeal bread (4 slices)

Wholemeal wraps (2 × 40 g)

Whole-wheat pasta (80 g)

1 × for this phase:

Black olives (1 jar)

Fat-free broth

Pine nuts (1 bag)

Vanilla protein

Walnuts (1 bag)

Food substitutes

DRINKS

Coffee and tea (without sugar or milk), water.

BREAD & BREAKFAST

Muesli, porridge, Ready-brek, rice cake, wholemeal bread, wholemeal crisp bread.

STARCHY FOODS

Brown rice, couscous, potatoes, quinoa, sweet potatoes, wholewheat pasta.

DAIRY

Cheese (light), cheese spread (light), cottage cheese, low-fat Quark, low-fat yogurt, skimmed milk.

MEAT/POULTRY

Chicken breast, beef tartare, smoked beef, steak, turkey breast.

MEAT SUBSTITUTES

Eggs, lentils, kidney beans, Quorn, tofu, peas, soybeans, tempeh, tofu.

FISH

Eel, mackerel, salmon, shrimp (no more than 2 per week), trout, tuna, white fish (no batter or other coating)

SPREADS FOR BREAD

Beef tartare (10 g), cooked chicken breast, cottage cheese, fruit (apple slices, banana, strawberries), houmous, peanut butter, smoked beef, vegetables (cucumber, radish, tomato).

VEGETABLES

All types of vegetables are allowed, a minimum 200 g per person per day. Vegetables contain lots of fibre and there-fore aid digestion.

Asparagus, aubergine, beetroot, brassica, Brussel sprouts, carrots, courgette, cucumber, endive, green beans, leek, mushrooms, onions, peppers, radish, runner beans, spinach, tomatoes.

FRUIT

Apple, grapefruit, grapes, kiwi fruit, lemon, mango, melon, orange, peach, pineapple, pome-granate, red fruits (blue-berries, raspberries etc.), tangerine/mandarin.

FATS AND OILS

Avocado, butter, coconut oil, nuts (unsalted, unroasted), oily fish, olive oil.

Bibliography

NUTRITION

Henselmans 2015, http://bayesianbodybuilding.com/why-women-should-not-train-like-men

EAT TO LOSE FAT: REFEED!

Mark van Oosterwijck, *Vet Verliezen de Ultieme Strategie (The Ultimate Weight Loss Strategy)*.

Bubbico, A., & Kravitz, L. (2011). 'Muscle hypertrophy: New insights and training recommendations'. *Fitness Journal*, 2326.

HOW MUCH PROTEIN DO YOU NEED WHILE TRAINING?

Hoffman, J.R., Ratamess, N.A., Kang, J., Falvo, M.J., Faigenbaum, A.D. J Int Soc Sports Nutr. 2006 Dec 13; 3:12–8.

Tarnopolsky, M. A., Atkinson, S.A., MacDougall, J.D., Chesley, A., Phillips, S., & Schwarcz, H.P. (1992). 'Evaluation of protein requirements for trained strength athletes'. *Journal of Applied Physiology*, 73(5), 1986–1995. *Macronutrient content of a hypoenergy diet affects nitrogen retention and muscle function in weight lifters.*

Walberg, J.L., Leidy, M.K., Sturgill, D.J., Hinkle, D.E., Ritchey, S.J., Sebolt, D.R. Int J Sports Med. 1988 Aug; 9(4):261–6. *Protein requirements and muscle mass/strength changes during intensive training in novice bodybuilders.*

Lemon, P.W., Tarnopolsky, M.A., MacDougall, J.D., Atkinson, S.A. J Appl Physiol. 1992 Aug; 73(2): 767–75. *Influence of protein intake and training status on nitrogen balance and lean body mass.*

Tarnopolsky, M.A., MacDougall, J.D., Atkinson, S.A. J Appl Physiol. 1988 Jan; 64(1):187–93. *Dietary protein for athletes: From requirements to optimum adaptation.*

Phillips, S.M., Van Loon ,L.J.. J Sports Sci. 2011; 29 Suppl 1:S29-38. *Protein and amino acid metabolism during and after exercise and the effects of nutrition.*

Rennie, M.J., Tipton, K.D. Annu Rev Nutr. 2000; 20:457–83.

Hartman, J.W., Moore, D.R., & Phillips, S.M. (2006). *Resistance training reduces whole-body protein turnover and improves net protein retention in untrained young males. Applied Physiology, Nutrition and Metabolism,* 31, 557–564.

Moore, D.R., Del Bel, N.C., Nizi, K.I., Hartman, J.W., Tang, J.E., Armstrong, D. et al. (2007). *Resistance training reduces fasted- and fed-state leucine turnover and increases dietary nitrogen retention in previously untrained young men.* Journal of Nutrition, 137, 985–991. *Effects of exercise on dietary protein requirements. Lemon PW. Int J Sport.*

Nutr. 1998 Dec; 8(4):426–47. *Effects of high-calorie supplements on body composition and muscular strength following resistance training.*

Rozenek. R., Ward, P., Long, S., Garhammer, J.J. Sports Med Phys Fitness. 2002 Sep; 42(3):340–7. *Increased protein maintains nitrogen balance during exercise-induced energy deficit.*

Pikosky, M.A,. Smith, T.J., Grediagin, A., Castaneda-Sceppa, C., Byerley, L., Glickman, E.L., Young, A.J. Med Sci Sports Exerc. 2008 Mar; 40(3):505–12. *Dietary carbohydrate-to-fat ratio: influence on whole-body nitrogen retention, substrate utilization, and hormone response in healthy male subjects.*

McCargar, L.J., Clandinin, M.T., Belcastro AN, Walker, K. Am J Clin Nutr. 1989 Jun; 49(6):1169–78. *Macronutrient intakes as determinants of dietary protein and amino acid adequacy.* Millward, D.J. J. Nutr. June 1, 2004 vol. 134 no. 6 1588S–1596S.

Index